MW01029685

Fetal Monitoring

A Multidisciplinary Approach

Mosby's
POCKET GUIDE TO
Fetal Monitoring
A Multidisciplinary Approach
Sixth Edition

SUSAN MARTIN TUCKER, MSN, RN, PHN
Nursing and Health Care Consultant
Quality Management and Perinatal Systems
Windsor, California

LISA A. MILLER, CNM, JD
President, Perinatal Risk Management and Education Services
Certified Nurse Midwife, Saint Anthony Hospital
Chicago, Illinois

DAVID A. MILLER, MD
Professor, Clinical Obstetrics, Gynecology, and Pediatrics
Keck School of Medicine
University of Southern California;
Medical Director, CHLA-USC
Institute for Maternal Fetal Health
Children's Hospital Los Angeles
Los Angeles, California

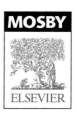

MOSBY

ELSEVIER

11830 Westline Industrial Drive
St. Louis, Missouri 63146

MOSBY'S POCKET GUIDE TO FETAL MONITORING: ISBN: 978-0-323-05670-0
A MULTIDISCIPLINARY APPROACH, SIXTH EDITION
Copyright © 2009 by Mosby, Inc., an affiliate of Elsevier Inc.

Notice

Knowledge and best practice in this field are constantly changing. As new research and experience broaden our knowledge, changes in practice, treatment and drug therapy may become necessary or appropriate. Readers are advised to check the most current information provided (i) on procedures featured or (ii) by the manufacturer of each product to be administered, to verify the recommended dose or formula, the method and duration of administration, and contraindications. It is the responsibility of the practitioner, relying on their own experience and knowledge of the patient, to make diagnoses, to determine dosages and the best treatment for each individual patient, and to take all appropriate safety precautions. To the fullest extent of the law, neither the Publisher nor the Authors assumes any liability for any injury and/or damage to persons or property arising out of or related to any use of the material contained in this book.

The Publisher

Previous editions copyrighted 2004, 2000, 1996, 1992, 1988

Library of Congress Cataloging-in-Publication Data
Tucker, Susan Martin, Date-
  Mosby's pocket guide to fetal monitoring : a multidisciplinary approach / Susan Martin Tucker, Lisa A. Miller, David A. Miller. -- 6th ed.
    p. ; cm.
  Rev. ed of: Pocket guide to fetal monitoring and assessment / Susan Martin Tucker. 5th ed. c2004.
  Includes bibliographical references and index.
  ISBN 978-0-323-05670-0 (pbk. : alk. paper) 1. Fetal monitoring--Handbooks, manuals, etc. 2. Fetal heart rate monitoring--Handbooks, manuals, etc. I. Miller, Lisa A. (Lisa Anne), Date-II. Miller, David A. (David Arthur), Date-III. Tucker, Susan Martin, Date-Pocket guide to fetal monitoring and assessment. IV. Title. V. Title: Pocket guide to fetal monitoring and assessment.
  [DNLM: 1. Fetal Monitoring--Handbooks. 2. Fetal Monitoring--Nurses' Instruction. 3. Fetal Diseases--diagnosis--Handbooks. 4. Fetal Diseases--diagnosis--Nurses' Instruction. WQ 39 T894m 2009]
  RG628.T83 2009
  618.3′2075--dc22
                                                                                    2008008752

Acquisitions Editor: Catherine Jackson
Senior Developmental Editor: Laurie K. Gower
Publishing Services Manager: Deborah Vogel
Project Manager: Brandilyn Tidwell
Design: Teresa McBryan

Working together to grow
libraries in developing countries

www.elsevier.com | www.bookaid.org | www.sabre.org

ELSEVIER   BOOK AID International   Sabre Foundation

Printed in the United States of America

Last digit is the print number: 9 8 7 6 5 4 3 2 1

CONTRIBUTOR

TEKOA KING, CNM, MPH, FACNM
Associate Clinical Professor
Department of Obstetrics, Gynecology, and Reproductive Services
University of California at San Francisco
San Francisco, California

REVIEWERS

SUZANNE McMURTRY BAIRD, MSN, RN
Assistant Professor, School of Nursing
Vanderbilt University
Nashville, Tennessee

HAYWOOD BROWN, MD
Professor and Chairman, OB/GYN
Duke University Medical Center
Durham, North Carolina

JAMES M. KELLEY, JD
Elk & Elk
Mayfield Heights, Ohio

LINDA FOWLER SHAHZAD, MSN, RNC
Clinical Nurse II, Women's Services
University of North Carolina Health Care
Chapel Hill, North Carolina

Clinical Computer Systems, Inc.
Elgin, Illinois

GE Medical Systems Information Technologies
Milwaukee, Wisconsin

Hill-Rom Company, Inc.
Batesville, Indiana

Philips Medical Systems
Böblingen, Germany

The new co-authors, Lisa A. Miller and David A. Miller, express
their deep gratitude to Susan Martin Tucker, who graciously
provided this opportunity for collaboration and teamwork
and upon whose strong foundation they are honored to build.

Welcome to the first multidisciplinary book on fetal monitoring, assessment, and management. The purpose of the sixth edition of *Pocket Guide to Fetal Monitoring: A Multidisciplinary Approach* is to provide a practical, portable, and evidence-based resource on fetal monitoring for all clinicians, whether nurse or physician, student or teacher. This edition, authored by a nurse, nurse-midwife, and a perinatologist, provides a truly multidisciplinary approach to fetal heart rate monitoring and fetal surveillance. Thoroughly revised to promote standardized nomenclature, standardized interpretation, and standardized management, this book offers clinicians the opportunity for effective collaboration in the management of fetal monitoring and assessment during both the antepartum and intrapartum periods.

DESCRIPTION

The goal of fetal heart rate monitoring is to prevent fetal injury that might result from disrupted fetal oxygenation during or prior to labor. Geared towards daily clinical practice, this book focuses on the application of evidence-based interpretation and management of fetal heart rate tracings in all settings. Beginning with a brief overview of the history of fetal monitoring, the book continues with information on the physiologic basis for monitoring, instrumentation for uterine and fetal heart rate monitoring, key factors in the evaluation of uterine activity, and fetal heart rate pattern identification using the standardized nomenclature developed by the National Institute of Child Health and Human Development (NICHD). An evidence-based method to interpretation and management is clearly outlined, and the influence of gestational age on fetal heart rate is discussed, along with the evaluation of fetal status outside the obstetric unit and in the antenatal setting. Throughout the text, a multidisciplinary patient safety approach is stressed, with an entire chapter devoted to documentation and risk management.

FEATURES

Some of the unique features of this book are:
- Content follows a logical and progressive sequence with *advanced* concepts to augment the information base for the

experienced clinician and *basic* elements to provide the foundation in fetal monitoring for those who are new to the subject matter.

■ The liberal use of tables, charts, and graphs makes it easy to locate and access key information, such as the oxygen pathway and fetal response to hypoxemia, interpretation of fetal heart rate patterns, and standardized management schematics.

■ Illustrative fetal monitor strips and other figures are included for their educational value to support and supplement the content.

■ Evidence levels are provided for information regarding various fetal heart rate patterns, and several common obstetric myths are laid to rest.

ORGANIZATION

Chapter 1 provides an overview of the history of fetal monitoring. It includes information on the development of the NICHD terminology as well as information on the future of electronic fetal monitoring and new developments such as ST analysis.

Chapter 2 discusses the physiologic basis for monitoring. Outlining the flow of oxygen from the environment to the fetus, it introduces the concept of the oxygen pathway, and provides the framework for evaluation of the fetal response to hypoxia. The mechanism of fetal injury due to hypoxic-ischemic encephalopathy is reviewed, including the criteria necessary to link intrapartum events with such injury.

Chapter 3 covers instrumentation for both auscultation and electronic fetal monitoring and provides step-by-step procedures with rationales for the application of monitoring devices. Information is presented on artifact detection, troubleshooting the monitor, telemetry with waterproof transducers (for patients in bed, ambulating, or in the bath), and computer-based systems (with central stations, analysis/alert capability, and data storage). Additionally, it includes information on the newest adjunct to electronic fetal monitoring, the ST waveform analyzer (STAN®; Neoventa Medical, Göteborg, Sweden).

Chapter 4 presents detailed information on uterine activity evaluation with a discussion of both normal and excessive uterine activity, the diagnosis and management of abnormal labor patterns, and the link between excessive uterine activity and fetal acidemia. A discussion of risk management issues related to oxytocin use is included.

Chapter 5 introduces the three separate but interdependent elements necessary for clinical practice: terminology, interpretation, and management. Definitions based on those of the NICHD are reviewed, along with underlying physiology and clinical significance. Definitions are accompanied by illustrations to assist the clinician in recognition of the nomenclature. Additionally, many patterns and terms that were not defined by the NICHD are illustrated and discussed using an evidence-based approach.

Chapter 6 presents a clear, concise, and systematic approach to the management of fetal heart rate tracings based on fetal oxygenation and response to hypoxemia. This comprehensive approach addresses all five essential components of a FHR tracing together: baseline rate, variability, accelerations, presence or absence of decelerations, and changes or trends in the tracing over time. It elucidates the *primary objective* of intrapartum FHR monitoring: to prevent fetal injury that might result from disrupted fetal oxygenation during labor.

Chapter 7 discusses the influence of gestational age on the interpretation of fetal heart rate. Maturational factors and behavioral states may result in unique responses in the fetal heart rate tracings of the preterm fetus and the postterm fetus. A discussion of management issues that arise during both antepartum and intrapartum monitoring is included.

Chapter 8 presents options for performing fetal assessment in the non-obstetric setting—for example, during transport, when associated with trauma, emergency services, and during non-obstetric surgical procedures. A sample triage tool is provided for managing the pregnant patient in the emergency department, and a decision tree is provided for managing the unstable pregnant trauma victim. In addition, physiologic adaptations to pregnancy are listed to avoid their being interpreted as pathologic, which they indeed might be in the nonpregnant woman.

Chapter 9 presents biophysical and biochemical methods of antepartum testing, including the nonstress test, the contraction stress test, vibroacoustic stimulation, ultrasound, the biophysical profile, an algorithm for antepartum testing, and fetal lung maturity tests.

Chapter 10 includes current information on patient safety, risk management, and documentation. Human error, common errors in perinatal units, and characteristics of high-reliability units are reviewed, and a systematic approach to patient safety is illustrated with a case study. Documentation issues and legal implications related to electronic fetal monitoring are addressed, including excerpts of actual deposition testimony related to documentation. Electronic record-keeping and new advances in data review are examined, and risk management strategies are summarized.

Appendix B is provided for colleagues outside of North America who monitor patients at a paper speed of 1 cm/min, as contrasted with the faster 3 cm/min speed used primarily in North America.

Pocket Guide to Fetal Monitoring: A Multidisciplinary Approach was written by clinicians, for clinicians. It is intended for use by nurses, nurse-midwives, medical students, physicians, resident physicians, clinical specialists, educators, and risk management and medical-legal professionals who have a theoretical background in obstetrics. In addition, the format provides essential concepts in a clear, concise, and easily understandable manner for those who are new to fetal monitoring/cardiotocography.

SUSAN MARTIN TUCKER

LISA A. MILLER

DAVID A. MILLER

CONTENTS

CHAPTER 1

A Brief History of Fetal Monitoring

"From the changes occurring in strength and rate of fetal heart beats, wouldn't it be possible to know about the status of health or sickness of the fetus?"
(Le Jumeau JA, 1822, quoted by Sureau[33])

Approximately 4 million women give birth each year in the United States. The majority of these women (85%) have continuous electronic fetal monitoring during labor.[26] Yet intrapartum fetal heart rate monitoring has not led to a significant reduction in neonatal neurologic morbidity.[31] Furthermore, early randomized trials and meta-analyses indicated that women who have continuous electronic fetal monitoring during labor have higher cesarean section rates than women who don't have continuous electronic fetal monitoring.[1] The reason this conundrum exists is a story that began nearly 200 years ago.

HISTORICAL OVERVIEW

Fetal heart tones were first heard in the seventeenth century. Jean Alexandre Le Jumeau, Vicomte de Kergaradec, used a stethoscope hoping to hear the noise of the water in the uterus and identified the noise he heard as the fetal heart rate. Le Jumeau was the first person to speculate in print about potential clinical uses for fetal heart rate auscultation.[33]

Early clinical use of determining the presence or absence of fetal heart sounds included confirmation of pregnancy, identification of twin gestation, and justification for a postmortem cesarean section. In 1833 William Kennedy, a British obstetrician, published a description of "fetal distress" by describing what would later be identified as a late deceleration. Kennedy correctly associated late decelerations with poor prognosis, and he made the link between fetal head compression and fetal bradycardia.[21] Other discoveries from early use of fetal heart rate assessment via intermittent auscultation included identification of fetal tachycardia in response to

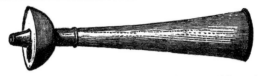

FIGURE 1-1 Early obstetric trumpet stethoscope. (Courtesy Wellcome Library, London.)

maternal fever, fetal heart rate decelerations following excessive uterine activity, and accelerations accompanying fetal movement (Figure 1-1).[33]

In 1917 the head stethoscope, or DeLee-Hillis fetoscope, was first reported in the literature.[16] During the 1950s, physicians, including Edward Hon[17-19] in the United States, Caldeyro-Barcia[7] in Uruguay, and Hammacher[13] in Germany, developed electronic devices that were able to continuously measure and record the fetal heart rate and uterine activity. The simultaneous measurement of fetal heart rate and uterine activity came to be called electronic fetal monitoring or cardiotocography. This new technologic capability permitted systematic study of the relationships between recorded fetal heart rate patterns and fetal physiology.[18,19,22] Investigators throughout the world made similar observations of fetal heart rate characteristics but developed different terms and definitions (Figure 1-2).

RANDOMIZED TRIALS OF ELECTRONIC FETAL MONITORING

In the 1960s observational studies demonstrated a decrease in intrapartum stillbirth rates in settings that adopted continuous electronic fetal monitoring.[10,26,29,38] These findings fueled widespread adoption of the technology into clinical practice. Although electronic fetal monitoring was originally intended for use in high-risk laboring women, it was rapidly incorporated into the management of low-risk laboring women as well.

In the 1970s several randomized clinical trials were conducted comparing continuous electronic fetal monitoring with intermittent auscultation using a Pinard stethoscope or a hand-held Doppler device.* Continuous electronic fetal monitoring was not associated

---

*14-16,20,21,24,25,26,29,32,33,36,38

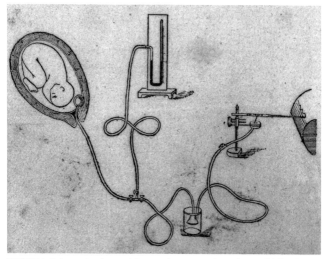

FIGURE 1-2 Apparatus for studying uterine contractions during childbirth. (Courtesy Wellcome Library, London.)

with a decrease in low Apgar scores or perinatal mortality. However, there was an increase in the incidence of cesarean section in women who had continuous electronic fetal monitoring. Despite these findings, use of continuous electronic fetal monitoring did not decrease, and by the 1990s its use had become nearly ubiquitous.

Meta-analyses have reviewed the results of trials comparing continuous intrapartum electronic fetal monitoring to intermittent auscultation.[1,34,35] These studies included over 37,000 women. Compared to intermittent auscultation, continuous electronic fetal monitoring showed no significant difference in overall perinatal death, but was associated with a significant reduction in neonatal seizures. No significant difference was detected in the incidence of cerebral palsy. However, there was a significant increase in cesarean sections associated with continuous electronic fetal monitoring. Interestingly, none of the randomized trials published after 1980 demonstrated a statistically significant increase in the rate of cesarean section in electronically monitored patients. More importantly, the majority of newborns in the cohort who later developed cerebral palsy were not in the group of fetuses who had fetal heart rate tracings that were considered "ominous."[12]

FETAL HEART RATE MONITORING RESEARCH AT THE END OF THE TWENTIETH CENTURY

What went wrong? Several things. Although the randomized controlled trials followed the usual guidelines for inclusion and exclusion of subjects and used recommended methods for the study protocols, the definitions of fetal heart rate patterns reflecting "fetal distress" varied among the different studies.[24,28,37] In addition, many of the studies were conducted before the importance of fetal heart rate variability, a critical parameter, was recognized. Finally, the outcome measures (Apgar scores, perinatal mortality, cerebral palsy) were nonspecific indicators of intrapartum asphyxia. As a result, the conclusions of these studies remain open to alternative interpretations.[30,36]

During the last half of the 1990s, an expert panel was convened to review the literature and make recommendations about the relationship between fetal heart rate patterns and intrapartum asphyxia. In 1996 the National Institute of Child Health and Human Development (NICHD) Task Force met and made recommendations[27] for three important aspects of fetal heart rate monitoring for both research and clinical practice: (1) The task force developed standard definitions for fetal heart rate patterns; (2) they described the fetal heart rate pattern (normal baseline rate, moderate variability, presence of accelerations, and absence of decelerations) that consistently reflects an absence of asphyxia; and (3) they described fetal heart rate patterns (recurrent late or variable decelerations or substantial bradycardia with absent variability) that are "predictive of current or impending asphyxia."

FETAL ASSESSMENT AT THE BEGINNING OF THE TWENTY-FIRST CENTURY

The NICHD definitions have been increasingly used in research investigating the relationship between fetal heart rate patterns and fetal acidemia, and they have been endorsed for daily clinical use by the American College of Obstetricians and Gynecologists[3] (ACOG), the Association of Women's Health, Obstetric, and Neonatal Nurses[6] (AWHONN), and the American College of Nurse-Midwives[2] (ACNM). Yet despite the use of standardized terminology, fetal heart rate monitoring continues to be an imprecise measure of fetal acidemia, and abnormal fetal heart rate patterns are relatively inaccurate predictors of poor newborn outcome.[31]

In 2003, the Task Force on Neonatal Encephalopathy and Cerebral Palsy[4] was convened by ACOG to review the world literature regarding the relationship between fetal heart rate patterns in labor and neonatal outcomes. The task force reviewed the literature on Apgar scores, neonatal encephalopathy and cerebral palsy, neonatal seizures, and umbilical cord gases. The task force identified clinical criteria necessary to define an acute intrapartum hypoxic event as sufficient to cause cerebral palsy. The report is discussed in detail in Chapter 2.

In an effort to find a more direct measure of fetal oxygenation to serve as an adjunct to electronic fetal monitoring in the assessment of fetal acid/base balance, fetal pulse oximetry made a short-lived appearance on the clinical scene. The first randomized trial of fetal pulse oximetry demonstrated a reduction in the number of cesarean sections performed for "nonreassuring" fetal heart rate patterns but no overall reduction in cesarean section.[11] At the time of this writing, fetal pulse oximetry has been a useful tool for research but is no longer available for use in clinical practice.

Outside the United States, computer analysis of the fetal electrocardiogram ST segment (STAN®; Neoventa Medical, Göteborg, Sweden) is being used as an adjunct to electronic fetal monitoring for pregnancies that are 36 weeks of gestation or greater.[5] ST wave-form analysis requires a specialized internal scalp electrode and monitor. The technology is based on evaluation of the ST segment and the T/QRS ratio of the fetal electrocardiogram complex, which are influenced by myocardial hypoxia. The goal of the technology is to prevent development of significant metabolic acidemia in the fetus by providing clinicians with an early warning of changes indicative of impending metabolic acidemia, thereby promoting timely intervention. STAN® technology is discussed further in Chapters 3 and 6.

What began in 1822 with a stethoscope has evolved into a complex technology that often provides as many questions as answers. Clinicians today have access to peer-reviewed professional journals, professional guidelines, and many excellent resources on fetal monitoring. Yet providers and consumers continue to debate the advantages and limitations of widespread use of electronic fetal monitoring. Consumers often read general news publications about the incidence of false alarms and subsequent cesarean sections with electronic fetal monitoring.[8,9] Clinicians repeatedly conclude that more research is needed on electronic fetal monitoring reliability (observer agreement), validity (association with neonatal outcomes), and efficacy (preventive interventions that work). Clearly, additional research is needed to further our knowledge of intrapartum fetal acidemia and to refine our ability to assess the fetus during labor.

In the future, care providers will need collaborative strategies for integrating increasingly complex biotechnologies and information technologies into best practices. Clinicians must recognize the features of the electronic fetal monitoring tracing that provide information regarding the absence of fetal metabolic acidemia, as demonstrated by the presence of accelerations and moderate variability, and must respond appropriately when those signs are absent. Standardization of terminology, multidisciplinary education regarding fetal heart rate interpretation and underlying physiology, and management based on collaboration and teamwork remain the best approaches to safe passage for mother and child, regardless of the technology employed.

References

1. Alfirevic Z, Devane D, Gyte GML: Continuous cardiotocography (CTG) as a form of electronic fetal monitoring (EFM) for fetal assessment during labour. *Cochrane Database Syst Rev* 3:CD006066, 2006. DOI: 10.1002/14651858.

2. American College of Nurse-Midwives: *Standard Nomenclature for Electronic Fetal Monitoring. Position Statement 2006.* Silver Spring, MD, 2006, ACNM.

3. American College of Obstetricians and Gynecologists: Intrapartum fetal heart rate monitoring, *Practice Bulletin* no. 62, 2005. *Obstet Gynecol* 106(6):1453-1460, 2006.

4. American College of Obstetricians and Gynecologists Task Force on Neonatal Encephalopathy and Cerebral Palsy, American Academy of Pediatrics: *Neonatal encephalopathy and cerebral palsy: Defining the pathogenesis and pathophysiology.* Washington, DC, 2003, ACOG, AAP.

5. Amer-Wåhlin I, Hellsten C, Norén H, Hagberg H, Herbst A, Kjellmer I, Lilja H, Lindoff C, Månsson M, Mårtensson L, Olofsson P, Sundström A, Marsál K: Cardiotocography only versus cardiotocography plus ST analysis of fetal electrocardiogram for intrapartum fetal monitoring A Swedish randomized controlled trial. *Lancet* 358(9281):534-538, 2001.

6. Association of Women's Health, Obstetric and Neonatal Nurses: *Changes to the FHMPP program.* Accessed August 22, 2005, from www.awhonn.org/awhonn/?pg=873-2180-17530.

7. Caldeyro-Barcia R, Mendez-Bauer C, Poseiro J, Escarcena L, Pose S, Bieniarz J, Arnt I, Gulin L, Althabe O: Control of human fetal heart rate during labor. In Cassels D, editor: *The heart and circulation in the newborn and infant.* New York, 1966, Grune & Stratton.

8. Cronin B: Health report: The bad news, *Time*, 35, March 18, 1996.
9. Declercq ER, Sakala C, Corry MP, Applebaum S: *Listening to mothers II: Report of the Second National U.S. Survey of Women's Childbearing Experiences.* New York: Childbirth Connection, October 2006. Accessed January 31, 2008 from www.childbirthconnection.org/listeningtomothers/.
10. Erkkola R, Gronroos M, Punnonen R, Kilkku P: Analysis of intrapartum fetal deaths: Their decline with increasing electronic fetal monitoring. *Acta Obstet Gynecol Scand* 63(5):459-462, 1984.
11. Garite TJ, Dildy GA, McNamara H, Nageotte MP, Boehm FH, Dellinger EH, Knuppel RA, Porreco RP, Miller HS, Sunderji S, Varner MW, Swedlow DB: A multicenter controlled trial of fetal pulse oximetry in the intrapartum management of nonreassuring fetal heart rate patterns. *Am J Obstet Gynecol* 183(5):1049-1058, 2000.
12. Grant S, O'Brien N, Joy MT, Hennessy E, MacDonald D: Cerebral palsy among children born during the Dublin randomized trial of intrapartum monitoring. *Lancet* 2:1233-1235, 1989.
13. Hammacher K: New method for the selective registration of the fetal heart beat. *German Geburtshilfe Frauenheilkd* 22:1542-1543, 1962.
14. Havercamp AD, Orleans M, Langerdoerfer S, McFee J, Murphy J, Thompson HE: A controlled trial of differential effects of intrapartum fetal monitoring. *Am J Obstet Gynecol* 134(4):399-408, 1979.
15. Havercamp AD, Thompson HE, McFee JG, Cetrulo C: The evaluation of continuous fetal heart rate monitoring in high risk pregnancy. *Am J Obstet Gynecol* 125(3):310-320, 1976.
16. Hillis DS: Attachment for the stethoscope. *JAMA* 68:910, 1917.
17. Hon EH: Instrumentation of fetal heart rate and electrocardiography II. A vaginal electrode. *Am J Obstet Gynecol* 83:772, 1963.
18. Hon EH: The classification of fetal heart rate. I. A working classification. *Obstet Gynecol* 22:137-146, 1963.
19. Hon EH: The electronic evaluation of the fetal heart rate. *Am J Obstet Gynecol* 75:1215, 1958.
20. Kelso IM, Parsons RJ, Lawrence GF, Arora SS, Edmonds DK, Cooke ID: An assessment of continuous fetal heart rate monitoring in labor. *Am J Obstet Gynecol* 131(5):526-532, 1978.
21. Kennedy E: *Observations of obstetrical auscultation*, p. 311, Dublin, 1833, Hodges & Smith.
22. Lee ST, Hon EH: Fetal hemodynamic response to umbilical cord compression. *Obstet Gynecol* 22:553-562, 1963.
23. Leveno J, Cunningham FG, Nelson S, Roark M, Williams ML, Guzick D, Dowling S, Rosenfeld CR, Buckley A: A prospective comparison of selective and universal electronic fetal monitoring in 34,995 pregnancies. *N Engl J Med* 315(10):615-641, 1986.
24. Luthy DA, Shy KK, van Belle G, Larson EB, Hughes JP, Benedetti TJ, Brown ZA, Effer S, King JF, Stenchever MA: A randomized trial of electronic monitoring in preterm labor. *Obstet Gynecol* 69(5):687-695, 1987.

25. MacDonald D, Grant A, Sheridan-Pereira M, Boylan P, Chalmers I: The Dublin randomized controlled trial of intrapartum fetal heart rate monitoring. *Am J Obstet Gynecol* 152(5):524-539, 1985.

26. Martin JA, Hamilton BE, Sutton PD, Ventura SJ, Menacker F, Munson ML: Births: Final data for 2002. *Natl Vital Stat Rep* 2003 52(10):1-113.

27. National Institute of Child Health and Human Development Research Planning Workshop. Electronic fetal heart rate monitoring; Research guidelines for interpretation. *Am J Obstet Gynecol* 177(6):1385-1390, 1997; *J Obstet Gynecol Neonatal Nurs* 26(6):635–640, 1997.

28. Neldam S, Osler M, Hansen PK, Nim J, Smith SF, Hertel J: Intrapartum fetal heart rate monitoring in a combined low- and high-risk population: A controlled trial. *Eur J Obstet Gynecol Reprod Biol* 23(1-2):1-11, 1986.

29. Parer JT: Fetal heart rate monitoring. *Lancet* 2(8143):632-633, 1979.

30. Parer JT, King T: Whither fetal heart rate monitoring? *Obstet Gynecol Fertil* 22(5):149-192, 1999.

31. Parer JT, King TL, Flanders S, Fox M, Kilpatrick SJ: Fetal acidemia and electronic fetal heart rate patterns: Is there evidence of an association? *J Matern Fetal Neonatal Med* 19(5):289-294, 2006.

32. Renou P, Chang A, Anderson I, Wood C: Controlled trial of fetal intensive care. *Am J Obstet Gynecol* 126(4):470-745, 1976.

33. Sureau C: Historical perspectives: Forgotten past, unpredictable future. *Baillieres Clin Obstet Gynaecol* 10:167-184, 1996.

34. Thacker SB, Stroup DF, Peterson HB: Efficacy and safety of intrapartum electronic fetal monitoring: An update. *Obstet Gynecol* 86(4 Pt 1): 613-620, 1995.

35. Vintzileos AM, Nochimson DJ, Guzman ER, Knuppel RA, Lake M, Schifrin BS: Intrapartum electronic fetal heart rate monitoring versus intermittent auscultation: A meta-analysis. *Obstet Gynecol* 85:149-155, 1995.

36. Winkler CL, Hauth JC, Tucker JM, Owen J, Brumfield CG.: Neonatal complications at term as related to the degree of umbilical artery acidemia. *Am J Obstet Gynecol* 164(2):637-641, 1991.

37. Wood C, Renou P, Oats J, Farrell E, Beischer N, Anderson I: A controlled trial of fetal heart rate monitoring in a low risk obstetric population. *Am J Obstet Gynecol* 141(5):527-534, 1981.

38. Yeh SY, Diaz F, Paul RH: Ten-year experience of intrapartum fetal monitoring in Los Angeles County/University of Southern California Medical Center. *Am J Obstet Gynecol* 143(5):496-500, 1982.

CHAPTER 2

Physiologic Basis for Monitoring

The objective of intrapartum fetal heart rate (FHR) monitoring is to prevent fetal injury that might result from disruption of normal fetal oxygenation during labor. The underlying assumption is that disruption of fetal oxygenation leads to characteristic physiologic changes that can be detected by changes in the fetal heart rate. Understanding the physiologic basis for electronic fetal heart rate monitoring requires a realistic appraisal of this basic assumption. The role of intrapartum fetal heart rate monitoring in assessing the fetal physiologic changes caused by disrupted oxygenation can be summarized as follows:

1. Fetal oxygenation consists of two basic elements:
   - Transfer of oxygen from the environment to the fetus
   - The subsequent fetal response
2. Certain FHR patterns provide reliable information regarding both of the basic elements of fetal oxygenation.

This chapter reviews the physiology underlying fetal oxygenation, including transfer of oxygen from the environment to the fetus and the subsequent fetal response. The relationship between fetal oxygenation and fetal heart rate patterns is discussed later, in Chapters 5 and 6.

TRANSFER OF OXYGEN FROM ENVIRONMENT TO FETUS

Oxygen is carried from the environment to the fetus by maternal and fetal blood along a pathway that invariably includes the maternal lungs, heart, vasculature, uterus, placenta, and umbilical cord. The oxygen pathway from the environment to the fetus, illustrated in Figure 2-1, is a central concept in fetal heart rate monitoring. Disruption of normal oxygen transfer can occur at any or all of the points along the oxygen pathway. Therefore, it is essential to understand the physiology and pathophysiology involved in each step.

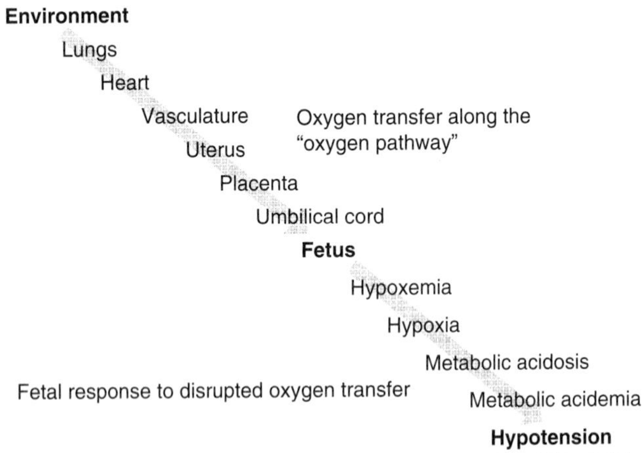

Environment
　　Lungs
　　　Heart
　　　　Vasculature　　Oxygen transfer along the
　　　　　Uterus　　　　"oxygen pathway"
　　　　　　Placenta
　　　　　　　Umbilical cord
　　　　　　　Fetus
　　　　　　　　Hypoxemia
　　　　　　　　　Hypoxia
　　　　　　　　　　Metabolic acidosis
Fetal response to disrupted oxygen transfer　Metabolic acidemia
　　　　　　　　　　Hypotension

FIGURE 2-1 Physiology of fetal oxygenation. (Courtesy David A. Miller, MD.)

External Environment

Oxygen makes up approximately 21% of inspired air. Therefore, in inspired air, the partial pressure exerted by oxygen gas is approximately 21% of total atmospheric pressure (760 mm Hg) minus the pressure exerted by water vapor (47 mm Hg). At sea level, this translates to approximately 150 mm Hg. As oxygen is transferred from the environment to the fetus, the partial pressure steadily declines. By the time oxygen reaches fetal umbilical venous blood, the partial pressure is as low as 30 mm Hg. After oxygen is delivered to fetal tissues, the PO_2 of deoxygenated blood in the umbilical arteries returning to the placenta is in the range of 15 to 25 mm Hg.[4-7] The sequential transfer of oxygen from the environment to the fetus and potential causes of disruption at each step are described below.

Maternal Lungs

Inspiration carries oxygenated air from the external environment to the distal air sacs of the lung, the alveoli. On the way to the alveoli, inspired air is diluted with carbon dioxide and less oxygenated air leaving the lungs. As a result, the PO_2 of air within the alveoli is significantly lower than that in inspired air. At sea level, normal alveolar PO_2 is in the range of 105 mm Hg. Disruption of normal oxygen transfer from the environment to the alveoli can result from upper airway obstruction or from disruption of breathing caused by depression of central respiratory control (narcotics, magnesium sulfate, seizure). From the alveoli, oxygen diffuses across a thin barrier into the pulmonary capillary blood. The pulmonary blood-gas barrier is made up of three layers: a single-cell layer of alveolar epithelium, a layer of extracellular collagen matrix (interstitium), and a single-cell layer of pulmonary capillary endothelium. Disruption of normal oxygen transfer from the alveoli to the pulmonary capillary blood can be caused by a number of factors, including ventilation-perfusion mismatch and diffusion defects. In an obstetric population, common pulmonary causes of disrupted oxygenation include respiratory depression due to medication or seizure, pulmonary embolus, pulmonary edema, pneumonia, asthma, atelectasis, and adult respiratory distress syndrome.

Maternal Blood

After diffusing from the pulmonary alveoli into maternal blood, more than 98% of oxygen combines with hemoglobin in maternal red blood cells. Approximately 1% to 2% remains dissolved in the blood and is measured by the partial pressure of dissolved oxygen (PaO_2). The amount of oxygen bound to hemoglobin depends directly upon the PaO_2. Hemoglobin saturations at various PaO_2 levels are illustrated by the oxyhemoglobin dissociation curve (Figure 2-2).

A normal adult PaO_2 value of 95 to 100 mm Hg results in hemoglobin saturation of approximately 95% to 98%, indicating that hemoglobin is carrying 95% to 98% of the total amount of oxygen it is capable of carrying. A number of factors affect the affinity of hemoglobin for oxygen and can shift the oxyhemoglobin dissociation curve to the left or right. In general, the tendency for hemoglobin to release oxygen is increased by factors that signal an increased requirement for oxygen. Specifically, oxygen release is enhanced by factors that indicate active cellular metabolism. These factors shift the oxyhemoglobin saturation curve to the right and include anaerobic glycolysis (reflected by increased 2,3-DPG concentration), production of hydrogen ions (reflected by decreased pH), and heat. Disruption of oxygen transfer from the environment to the fetus due to abnormal maternal oxygen carrying capacity can result from severe anemia or from hereditary or acquired abnormalities affecting oxygen binding (hemoglobinopathies, methemoglobinemia). In an obstetric population, reduced maternal oxygen carrying capacity

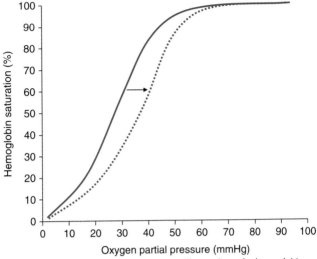

FIGURE 2-2 Fetal oxygen dissociation curve. The tendency for hemoglobin to release oxygen is increased by factors that signal an increased requirement for oxygen. Specifically, oxygen release is enhanced by factors that indicate active cellular metabolism. These factors shift the oxyhemoglobin saturation curve to the right and include anaerobic glycolysis (reflected by increased 2, 3-DPG concentration), production of hydrogen ions (reflected by decreased pH), and heat. (Courtesy David A. Miller, MD.)

rarely interferes with fetal oxygenation. Maternal hemoglobin saturation can be estimated non-invasively by transmission pulse oximetry (SpO_2). In recent years, investigators studying the efficacy of fetal oxygen saturation ($FSpO_2$) monitoring have provided valuable insights into fetal physiology (see Chapter 6).

Maternal Heart

From the lungs, pulmonary veins carry oxygenated maternal blood to the heart. Blood enters the left atrium with a PaO_2 of approximately 95 mm Hg. Oxygenated blood passes from the left atrium, through the mitral valve into the left ventricle and out the aorta for systemic distribution. Normal transfer of oxygen from the environment to the fetus is highly dependent upon normal cardiac function, reflected by cardiac output. Cardiac output is the product of heart rate and stroke volume. Heart rate is determined by the following:

- Intrinsic cardiac pacemakers (sinoatrial node, atrioventricular node)
- The cardiac conduction system
- Autonomic regulation (sympathetic, parasympathetic)
- Humoral factors (catecholamines)
- Extrinsic factors (medications)
- Local factors (calcium, potassium)

Stroke volume is determined by preload, contractility, and afterload. *Preload* is the amount of stretch on myocardial fibers at the end of diastole when the ventricles are full of blood. It is determined by the volume of venous blood returning to the heart. *Contractility* is the force and speed with which myocardial fibers shorten during systole to expel blood from the heart. *Afterload* is the pressure that opposes the shortening of myocardial fibers during systole and usually is estimated by the systemic vascular resistance or systemic blood pressure.

Disruption of oxygen transfer from the environment to the fetus at the level of the maternal heart can be caused by any condition that reduces cardiac output, including the following:

- Altered heart rate (arrhythmia)
- Reduced preload (hypovolemia, compression of the inferior vena cava)
- Impaired contractility (ischemic heart disease, diabetes, cardiomyopathy, congestive heart failure)
- Increased afterload (hypertension)

In addition, structural abnormalities of the heart and/or great vessels may impede the normal ability to pump blood (valvular stenosis, valvular insufficiency, pulmonary hypertension, coarctation of the aorta). In a healthy obstetric patient, the most common cause of reduced cardiac output is reduced preload (hypovolemia, compression of the inferior vena cava).

Maternal Vasculature

Oxygenated blood leaving the heart is carried by the systemic vasculature to the uterus. The path includes the aorta, common iliac artery, internal iliac artery, anterior division of the internal iliac artery, and the uterine artery. From the uterine artery, oxygenated blood travels through the arcuate arteries, the radial arteries, and finally the spiral arteries before exiting the maternal vasculature and entering the intervillous space of the placenta. *Disruption of normal oxygen transfer from the environment to the fetus at the level of the maternal vasculature commonly results from hypotension* (for example, regional anesthesia, hypovolemia, impaired venous return, impaired cardiac output, medications). Alternatively, it may result from vasoconstriction of distal arterioles in response to endogenous vasoconstrictors or medications. Conditions associated with chronic vasculopathy, such as chronic hypertension, long-standing diabetes, collagen vascular disease, thyroid disease and renal disease, may result in chronic suboptimal transfer of oxygen and nutrients to the fetus. Preeclampsia is associated with abnormal vascular remodeling at the level of the spiral arteries and can impede normal perfusion of the intervillous space. Catastrophic vascular injury (trauma, aortic dissection) is rare. In a healthy obstetric patient, transient hypotension is the most common cause of disrupted oxygen transfer at this level.

Uterus

Between the maternal uterine arteries and the intervillous space of the placenta, the arcuate, radial, and spiral arteries traverse the muscular wall of the uterus. Disruption of normal oxygen transfer from the environment to the fetus at the level of the uterus commonly results from uterine contractions that compress intramural blood vessels and impede the flow of blood. *Excessive uterine activity and uterine injury (rupture, trauma) are the most common causes of acute disruption of fetal oxygenation at this level.* Uterine activity and its evaluation are discussed in Chapter 4.

Placenta

The placenta is the maternal-fetal interface that facilitates the exchange of gases, nutrients, wastes and other molecules (for example, antibodies, hormones, medications) between maternal blood in the intervillous space and fetal blood in the villous capillaries. On the maternal side of the placenta, oxygenated blood exits the spiral arteries and enters the intervillous space to surround and bathe the chorionic villi. On the fetal side of the placenta, paired umbilical arteries carry blood from the fetus through the umbilical cord to the placenta (Figure 2-3). At term, the umbilical arteries receive 40% of fetal cardiac output. Upon reaching the placental cord insertion site, the umbilical arteries divide into multiple branches and fan out across the surface of the placenta. At each cotyledon, placental arteries dive beneath the surface en route to the chorionic villi (Figure 2-4). The chorionic villi are thousands of tiny branches of

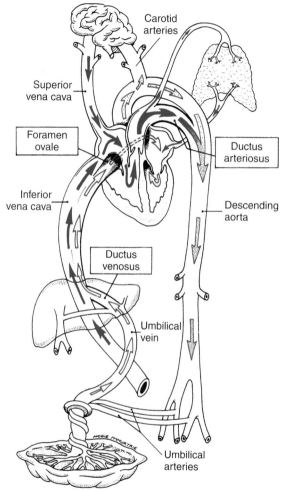

FIGURE 2-3 Fetal circulation. Oxygenated and nutrient-rich blood is carried to the fetus by the umbilical vein to the fetal heart. Oxygen-poor and waste product-rich blood circulates back to the placenta via the umbilical arteries. Three anatomic shunts (the ductus venosus, the foramen ovale, and the ductus arteriosus) permit fetal blood to bypass the liver and the lungs. (From Bloom RS: Delivery room resuscitation of the newborn. In Martin RJ, Fanaroff AA, Walsh MC, editors: *Fanaroff and Martin's neonatal-perinatal medicine: Diseases of the fetus and infant*, ed 8, Philadelphia, 2006, Mosby.)

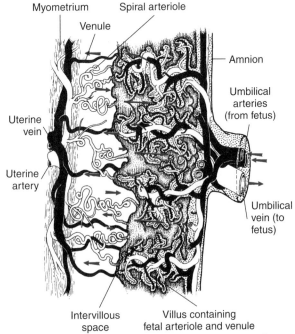

FIGURE 2-4 Schema of placenta. As maternal blood enters the intervillous space, it spurts from the uterine spiral arterioles and spreads laterally through the space. *White vessels* carry oxygenated blood. *Black vessels* carry oxygen-poor blood.

trophoblast that protrude into the intervillous space. Each branch of trophoblast is perfused by a fetal capillary bed that represents the terminal distribution of an umbilical artery. At term, fetal villous capillary blood is separated from maternal blood in the intervillous space by a thin blood-blood barrier similar to the blood-gas barrier in the maternal lung. The placental blood-blood barrier is made up of a layer of placental trophoblast and a layer of fetal capillary endothelium with intervening basement membranes and villous stroma. Substances are exchanged between maternal and fetal blood by a number of mechanisms, including simple (passive) diffusion, facilitated diffusion, active transport, bulk flow, pinocytosis, and leakage. These mechanisms are summarized in Table 2-1. Oxygen is transferred from the intervillous space to the fetal blood by a complex process that depends upon the PaO_2 of maternal blood perfusing the intervillous space, maternal blood flow within the intervillous

TABLE 2-1   Mechanisms of Exchange Between Fetal and Maternal Blood

Mechanism	Description	Substances
Simple diffusion	Passage of substances from a region of higher concentration to one of lower concentration along a concentration gradient that is passive and does not require energy	Oxygen Carbon dioxide Small ions (sodium chloride) Lipids Fat-soluble vitamins Many drugs
Facilitated diffusion	Passage of substances along a concentration gradient with the assistance of a carrier molecule involved	Glucose Carbohydrates
Active transport	Passage of substances against a concentration gradient; carrier molecules and energy are required	Amino acids Water-soluble vitamins Large ions
Bulk flow	Transfer of substances by a hydrostatic or osmotic gradient	Water Dissolved electrolytes
Pinocytosis	Transfer of minute, engulfed particles across a cell membrane	Immune globulins Serum proteins
Breaks and leakage	Small breaks in the placental membrane allowing passage of plasma and substances	Maternal or fetal blood cells (potentially resulting in isoimmunization)

space, chorionic villous surface area, and diffusion across the placental blood-blood barrier.

Intervillous Space PaO$_2$

As described previously, oxygenated maternal blood leaves the maternal heart with a PaO$_2$ of approximately 95 to 100 mm Hg. There are no capillary beds between the maternal heart and the spiral arteries; therefore, the oxygenated maternal blood exiting the spiral arteries and entering the intervillous space has a PaO$_2$ of approximately 95 to 100 mm Hg. Oxygen is released from maternal hemoglobin and diffuses across the placental blood-blood barrier into fetal blood where it combines with fetal hemoglobin. As a result, maternal blood in the intervillous space becomes relatively oxygen depleted and exits the intervillous space via uterine veins with a PaO_2 of approximately 40 mm Hg (Figure 2-5).

Therefore, the average PaO_2 of maternal blood in the intervillous space is between the PaO_2 of blood entering the intervillous space (95 to 100 mm Hg) and the PaO_2 of blood exiting the intervillous space (40 mm Hg). The average intervillous space PaO_2 is approximately 40 to 45 mm Hg. Disruption of normal fetal oxygenation can result from conditions that reduce the PaO_2 of maternal blood entering the intervillous space. These conditions were discussed previously.

Intervillous Space Blood Flow

At term, uterine perfusion accounts for 10% to 15% of maternal cardiac output, or approximately 700 to 800 mL per minute. Most of this blood is located in the intervillous space of the placenta surrounding the chorionic villi. Conditions that directly affect the volume of the intervillous space include collapse or destruction of the intervillous space due to placental abruption, infarction, thrombosis, or infection.

Chorionic Villous Surface Area

Optimal oxygen exchange requires normal chorionic villous surface area. Normal transfer of oxygen from the environment to the fetus at the level of the placenta can be disrupted by conditions that limit or reduce the chorionic villous surface area available for gas exchange. These conditions can be acute or chronic and include primary abnormalities in the development of the villous vascular tree

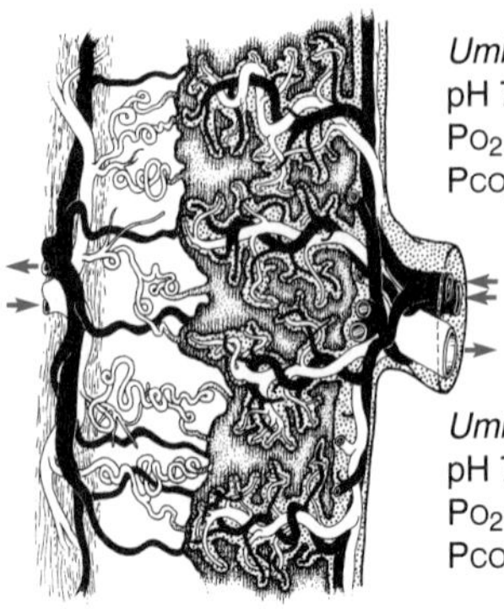

Uterine vein
pH 7.3
Po_2 40 mm Hg
Pco_2 40-50 mm Hg

Uterine artery
pH 7.4-7.45
Po_2 95-100 mm Hg
Pco_2 30-35 mm Hg

Umbilical arteries
pH 7.2-7.3
Po_2 15-25 mm Hg
Pco_2 45-55 mm Hg

Umbilical vein
pH 7.3-7.4
Po_2 25-35 mm Hg
Pco_2 35-45 mm Hg

FIGURE 2-5 Approximate maternal and fetal blood gas values.

or secondary destruction of normal chorionic villi by infarction, thrombosis, hemorrhage, inflammation, or infection.

Diffusion Across the Blood-Blood Barrier

Diffusion of a substance across the placental blood-blood barrier is dependent upon concentration gradient, molecular weight, lipid solubility, protein-binding, and ionization. In addition, diffusion rate is inversely proportional to diffusion distance. At term, the placental blood-blood barrier is very thin and the diffusion distance is short. Under normal circumstances, oxygen and carbon dioxide diffuse readily across this thin barrier. However, normal diffusion can be impeded by conditions that increase the distance between maternal and fetal blood. These conditions can be acute, subacute, or chronic and include villous hemorrhage, inflammation, thrombosis, infarction, edema, fibrosis, and excessive cellular proliferation (syncytial knots).[2,3,8]

Disruption of Placental Blood Vessels

Fetal blood loss caused by disruption of blood vessels at the level of the placenta warrants brief consideration. Damaged chorionic vessels can allow a significant amount of fetal blood to leak into the intervillous space, leading to fetal-maternal hemorrhage. This is often a consequence of abdominal trauma, but it can occur in association with placental abruption or invasive procedures. Ruptured vasa previa is a rare cause of fetal hemorrhage. Vasa previa is a placental vessel traversing the chorioamniotic membrane in close proximity to the cervical os. Such a vessel may be damaged by normal cervical change during labor or injured inadvertently during membrane rupture or digital exam.

Summary of Placental Causes of Disrupted Oxygenation

Although many conditions can interfere with the normal transfer of oxygen across the placenta, most involve the microvasculature and can be confirmed only by histopathology. Clinically, the most common cause of disrupted oxygen transfer at the level of the placenta is abruption or premature separation of placenta previa. Fetal-maternal hemorrhage and vasa previa should be considered in the appropriate clinical setting.

Fetal Blood

After oxygen has diffused from the intervillous space across the placental blood-blood barrier and into fetal blood, the PaO_2 is in the range of 30 mm Hg and fetal hemoglobin saturation is between 50% and 70%. Although fetal PaO_2 and hemoglobin saturation are low in comparison to adult values, adequate delivery of oxygen to the fetal tissues is maintained by a number of compensatory mechanisms. For example, fetal cardiac output per unit weight is three to four times greater than that of the adult. Hemoglobin concentration and affinity for oxygen are greater in the fetus as well, resulting in increased oxygen carrying capacity. Finally, oxygenated blood is directed preferentially toward vital organs by way of anatomic shunts at the level of the ductus venosus, foramen ovale, and ductus arteriosus. Conditions that can disrupt the normal transfer of oxygen from the environment to the fetus at the level of the fetal blood are uncommon but may include fetal anemia (alloimmunization, viral infections, fetal-maternal hemorrhage, vasa previa) and conditions that reduce oxygen carrying capacity (Bart's hemoglobinopathy, methemoglobinemia).

Umbilical Cord

After oxygen combines with fetal hemoglobin in the villous capillaries, oxygenated blood returns to the fetus by way of villous veins that coalesce to form placental veins on the surface of the placenta. Placental surface veins unite to form a single umbilical vein within the umbilical cord. Disruption of the normal transfer of oxygen from the environment to the fetus at the level of the umbilical cord most often results from simple mechanical compression. Other uncommon causes may include vasospasm, thrombosis, atherosis, hypertrophy, hemorrhage, inflammation, or a "true knot."

From the environment to the fetus, maternal and fetal blood carry oxygen along the oxygen pathway illustrated in Figure 2-1. Common causes of disrupted oxygen transfer at each step along the pathway are summarized in Table 2-2. In the interest of simplicity, the previous discussion was limited to one gas, oxygen. It is critical to note that gas exchange also involves the transfer of carbon dioxide in the opposite direction, that is, from the fetus to the environment. Any condition that disrupts the transfer of oxygen from the environment to the fetus has the potential to disrupt the transfer of carbon dioxide from the fetus to the environment. However, carbon dioxide diffuses across the placental blood-blood barrier more rapidly than does oxygen. Therefore, any disruption of the pathway is likely to impact oxygen transfer to a greater

TABLE 2-2 Some Causes of Disrupted Transfer of Oxygen from the Environment to the Fetus

Oxygen Pathway	Causes of Disrupted Oxygen Transfer
Lungs	Respiratory depression (narcotics, magnesium)
	Seizure (eclampsia)
	Pulmonary embolus
	Pulmonary edema
	Pneumonia/ARDS
	Asthma
	Atelectasis
	Rarely pulmonary hypertension
	Rarely chronic lung disease
Heart	Reduced cardiac output
	Hypovolemia
	Compression of the inferior vena cava
	Regional anesthesia (sympathetic blockade)
	Cardiac arrhythmia
	Rarely congestive heart failure
	Rarely structural cardiac disease
Vasculature	Hypotension
	Hypovolemia
	Compression of the inferior vena cava
	Regional anesthesia (sympathetic blockade)
	Medications (hydralazine, labetalol, nifedipine)
	Vasculopathy (chronic hypertension, SLE, preeclampsia)
	Vasoconstriction (cocaine, methylergonovine)
Uterus	Excessive uterine activity
	Uterine stimulants (prostaglandins, oxytocin)
	Uterine rupture
Placenta	Placental abruption
	Rarely vasa previa
	Rarely fetal–maternal hemorrhage
	Placental infarction, infection (usually confirmed retrospectively)
Umbilical cord	Cord compression
	Cord prolapse
	"True knot"

ARDS, adult respiratory distress syndrome; *SLE*, systemic lupus erythematosus.

extent than carbon dioxide transfer. As summarized previously, oxygen transfer from the environment to the fetus represents the first basic component of fetal oxygenation. The second basic component of fetal oxygenation involves the fetal physiologic response to disrupted oxygen transfer.

FETAL RESPONSE TO DISRUPTED OXYGEN TRANSFER

Depending upon frequency and duration, disruption of oxygen transfer at any point along the oxygen pathway may result in progressive deterioration of fetal oxygenation. The cascade begins with hypoxemia, defined as decreased oxygen content in the blood. At term, hypoxemia is characterized by an umbilical artery PaO_2 below the normal range of 15 to 25 mm Hg. Recurrent or sustained hypoxemia can lead to decreased delivery of oxygen to the tissues and reduced tissue oxygen content, or hypoxia. Normal homeostasis requires an adequate supply of oxygen and fuel in order to generate the energy required by basic cellular activities.

When oxygen is readily available, aerobic metabolism efficiently generates energy in the form of adenosine triphosphate. By-products of aerobic metabolism include carbon dioxide and water. When oxygen is in short supply, tissues may be forced to convert from aerobic to anaerobic metabolism, generating energy less efficiently and resulting in the production of lactic acid. Accumulation of lactic acid in the tissues results in metabolic acidosis. Lactic acid accumulation can lead to utilization of buffer bases (primarily bicarbonate) to help stabilize tissue pH. If the buffering capacity is exceeded, the blood pH may begin to fall, leading to metabolic acidemia. Eventually, recurrent or sustained tissue hypoxia and acidosis can lead to loss of peripheral vascular smooth muscle contraction, reduced peripheral vascular resistance, and hypotension.

Acidemia is defined as increased hydrogen ion content (decreased pH) in the blood. With respect to fetal physiology, it is critical to distinguish between respiratory acidemia, caused by accumulation of CO_2, and metabolic acidemia, caused by accumulation of fixed (lactic) acid. These distinct categories of acidemia have entirely different clinical implications and are discussed later in this chapter.

Mechanisms of Injury

If disrupted oxygen transfer progresses to the stage of metabolic acidemia and hypotension, as described earlier, multiple organs and systems (including the brain and heart) can suffer hypoperfusion, reduced oxygenation, lowered pH, and reduced delivery of fuel for metabolism. These changes can trigger a cascade of cellular events, including altered enzyme function, protease activation, ion shifts, altered water regulation, disrupted neurotransmitter metabolism, free radical production, and phospholipid degradation. Disruption of normal cellular metabolism can lead to cellular dysfunction, tissue dysfunction, and even death.

Injury Threshold

We have reviewed fetal oxygenation in detail, including each step of oxygen transfer from the environment to the fetus and each stage of the fetal physiologic response to disrupted oxygenation. Finally, we reviewed the mechanisms of injury in the setting of recurrent or sustained disruption of oxygenation. The relationship between disrupted fetal oxygenation and neurologic injury is complex. Electronic fetal heart rate monitoring was introduced with the expectation that it would significantly reduce the incidence of neurologic injury (specifically cerebral palsy) caused by intrapartum disruption of fetal oxygenation. In recent years, it has become apparent that most cases of cerebral palsy are unrelated to intrapartum events and therefore cannot be prevented by intrapartum fetal heart rate monitoring. Nevertheless, a significant minority of such cases may be related to intrapartum events and continue to generate controversy.

In January 2003, the American College of Obstetricians and Gynecologists and the American Academy of Pediatrics jointly published a monograph[1] titled "Neonatal Encephalopathy and Cerebral Palsy: Defining the Pathogenesis and Pathophysiology," summarizing the world literature regarding the relationship between intrapartum events and neurologic injury. Agencies and professional organizations that reviewed and endorsed the report include the Centers for Disease Control and Prevention, the Child Neurology Society, the March of Dimes Birth Defects Foundation, the National Institute of Child Health and Human Development, the Royal Australian and New Zealand College of Obstetricians and Gynecologists, the Society for Maternal-Fetal Medicine, and the Society of Obstetricians and Gynaecologists of Canada. The consensus report established four essential criteria defining an acute intrapartum event sufficient to cause cerebral palsy (Box 2-1).

The first criterion provides crucial information regarding the threshold of fetal injury in the setting of intrapartum disruption of oxygenation. Specifically, it indicates that intrapartum disruption of fetal oxygenation does not result in injury unless it progresses at least to the stage of significant metabolic acidemia (umbilical artery pH < 7.0 and base deficit ≥ 12 mmol/L). It is important to note that

BOX 2-1 Essential Criteria That Define an Acute Intrapartum Event Sufficient to Cause Cerebral Palsy*

1. Umbilical cord arterial blood pH <7.0 and base deficit ≥12 mmol/L
2. Early onset of moderate to severe neonatal encephalopathy in infants born at 34 or more weeks of gestation
3. Cerebral palsy of the spastic quadriplegic or dyskinetic type
4. Exclusion of other identifiable etiologies such as trauma, coagulation disorders, infectious conditions, or genetic disorders

*Must meet all four.

fetal injury is uncommon even when metabolic acidemia is present. It is also important to understand that respiratory acidemia is not a recognized risk factor for fetal injury. This information has significant implications for the interpretation and management of intrapartum fetal heart rate patterns, which are reviewed in Chapter 6.

The second criterion highlights an equally important point. Specifically, intrapartum disruption of fetal oxygenation does not result in cerebral palsy unless it first causes moderate to severe neonatal encephalopathy. The report further clarified that neonatal encephalopathy has many possible causes. Hypoxic-ischemic encephalopathy resulting from intrapartum disruption of fetal oxygenation represents only a small subset of the larger category of neonatal encephalopathy. The relationship among hypoxic-ischemic encephalopathy, neonatal encephalopathy, and cerebral palsy is illustrated in Figure 2-6.

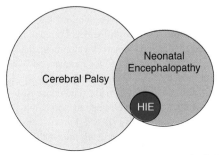

FIGURE 2-6 Relationship of hypoxic-ischemic encephalopathy (HIE) to neonatal encephalopathy and cerebral palsy. NOTE: HIE is a small subset of conditions that cause neonatal encephalopathy, which is a subset of conditions that cause cerebral palsy. (Courtesy Patricia R. McCartney, PhD, RNC.)

BOX 2-2   Criteria That Collectively Suggest Injury Occurred Within 48 Hours of Birth

1. A sentinel hypoxic event immediately before or during labor
2. A sudden and sustained fetal bradycardia or the absence of FHR variability in the presence of persistent late or variable decelerations, usually after a hypoxic sentinel event when the pattern was previously normal
3. Apgar scores of 0-3 beyond 5 minutes
4. Onset of multisystem involvement within 72 hours of birth

The third criterion emphasizes that different subtypes of cerebral palsy have different clinical origins. Spastic quadriplegia is associated with injury to the parasagittal cerebral cortex and involves abnormal motor control of all four extremities. The dyskinetic subtype of cerebral palsy is associated with injury to the basal ganglia and involves disorganized, choreoathetoid movements. The report concluded that these are the only two subtypes of cerebral palsy that are associated with *hypoxic-ischemic injury* in term and near-term pregnancies. Specifically, spastic diplegia, hemiplegia, ataxia, and hemiparetic cerebral palsy are "unlikely to result from acute intrapartum hypoxia." The report further concluded that other conditions, including epilepsy, mental retardation, and attention deficit hyperactivity disorder, do not result from birth asphyxia in the absence of cerebral palsy.

The fourth criterion underscores the fact that intrapartum hypoxic-ischemic injury is a potential factor in only a small subset of all cases of cerebral palsy. Most cases of cerebral palsy are unrelated to intrapartum events.

The report identified four additional criteria that can help establish the timing of injury, emphasizing that these criteria are "nonspecific to asphyxial insults" (Box 2-2).

SUMMARY

The physiology of fetal oxygenation involves the sequential transfer of oxygen from the environment to the fetus and the subsequent fetal response (see Figure 2-1). Although disruption of normal oxygen transfer can occur at any point along the oxygen pathway, examples of causes that might be encountered in a typical obstetric population are summarized in Table 2-2. Recurrent or sustained disruption of normal oxygen transfer can lead to progressive deterioration of fetal oxygenation and eventually to potential fetal injury. However, the joint consensus report by the American College of Obstetricians and Gynecologists and the American Academy of Pediatrics defined significant metabolic acidemia (umbilical artery pH < 7.0 and base deficit ≥12 mmol/L) as an essential pre-condition to intrapartum hypoxic injury.[1] With respect to the relationship between fetal oxygenation and potential injury, there is consensus in the literature that disrupted oxygenation does not result in fetal injury unless it progresses at least to the stage of significant metabolic acidemia.

The physiologic basis of fetal heart rate monitoring can be summarized in a few key concepts:

1. The objective of intrapartum FHR monitoring is to assess fetal oxygenation during labor.
2. Fetal oxygenation involves the transfer of oxygen from the environment to the fetus and the subsequent fetal response.
3. Oxygen is transferred from the environment to the fetus by maternal and fetal blood along a pathway that invariably includes the maternal lungs, heart, vasculature, uterus, placenta, and umbilical cord.
4. The fetal response to disrupted oxygen transfer involves the sequential progression from hypoxemia to hypoxia, metabolic acidosis, metabolic acidemia, and finally hypotension.
5. Fetal injury due to disrupted oxygenation does not occur unless this process has progressed at least to the stage of significant metabolic acidemia (umbilical artery pH <7.0 and base deficit >12 mmol/L).

Later chapters expand on these concepts as we discuss the interpretation and management of fetal heart rate patterns.

References

1. American College of Obstetricians and Gynecologists Task Force on Neonatal Encephalopathy and Cerebral Palsy, American College of Obstetricians and Gynecologists, American Academy of Pediatrics: *Neonatal encephalopathy and cerebral palsy: Defining the pathogenesis and pathophysiology.* Washington, DC, 2003, ACOG, AAP.
2. Arabin B, Jimenez E, Vogel M, Weitzel HK: Relationship of utero- and fetoplacental blood flow velocity wave forms with pathomorphological placental findings. *Fetal Diagn Ther* 7(3-4):173-179, 1992.
3. Giles WB, Trudinger BJ, Baird PJ: Fetal umbilical artery flow velocity waveforms and placental resistance: Pathological correlation. *Br J Obstet Gynaecol* 92(1):31-38, 1985.

4. Helwig JT, Parer JT, Kilpatrick SJ, Laros RK: Umbilical cord blood acid-base state: What is normal? *Am J Obstet Gynecol* 174(6):1807-1812, 1996.

5. Nodwell A, Carmichael L, Ross M, Richardson B: Placental compared with umbilical cord blood to assess fetal blood gas and acid-base status. *Obstet Gynecol* 105(1):129-138, 2005.

6. Richardson B, Nodwell A, Webster K, Alshimmiri M, Gagnon R, Natale R: Fetal oxygen saturation and fractional extraction at birth and the relationship to measures of acidosis. *Am J Obstet Gynecol* 178(3):572-579, 1998.

7. Victory R, Penava D, Da Silva O, Natale R, Richardson B: Umbilical cord pH and base excess values in relation to adverse outcome events for infants delivering at term. *Am J Obstet Gynecol* 191(6):2021-2028, 2004.

8. Trudinger B.: *Fetus and neonate: Physiology and clinical applications: The circulation*, pp. 323-338, Cambridge, United Kingdom, 1993, Cambridge University Press.

CHAPTER 3

Instrumentation for Fetal Heart Rate and Uterine Activity Monitoring

U terine activity (UA) and fetal heart rate (FHR) may be monitored by traditional (palpation and auscultation) or electronic means. Electronic fetal monitoring (EFM) can be accomplished using external or internal monitoring methods, or a combination of both. This chapter describes the devices and techniques used to monitor the fetal heart rate and uterine activity. Additionally, it includes information on telemetry, central displays, and the ST waveform analyzer (STAN®; Neoventa Medical, Göteborg, Sweden).

AUSCULTATION OF FETAL HEART RATE

Description

Auscultation of the fetal heart rate may be performed with a stethoscope, DeLee-Hillis fetoscope, Pinard stethoscope, or Doppler ultrasound (US) device (Figure 3-1). Auscultation is *not* simply electronic fetal monitoring without a tracing. While electronic fetal monitoring is based on visual assessment, auscultation is an *auditory* assessment in which an instrument or device is used to count the number of fetal heartbeats occurring in a prescribed amount of time. The rate obtained is utilized, along with other assessment data, to guide management and care of the maternal–fetal dyad.

If a *stethoscope* is used, the end should be turned to the domed, or bell, side of the stethoscope, rather than the flat side. The domed side is then placed on the maternal abdomen over the point of maximum intensity (PMI). The point of maximum intensity is the location where the fetal heart tones are heard the loudest, usually over the fetal back. The *fetoscope* should be applied to the listener's head, because bone conduction amplifies the fetal heart sounds for counting. It is the ventricular fetal heart sounds that can be counted

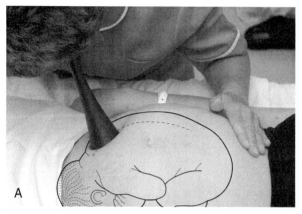

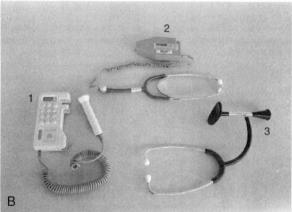

FIGURE 3-1 A. Auscultation of FHR with a Pinard stethoscope. Vertex left occipitoanterior. **B.** *1,* US fetoscope; *2,* US stethoscope; *3,* DeLee-Hillis fetoscope. (**A.** From Fraser DM, Cooper MA, editors: *Myles textbook for midwives,* ed 14, London, 2003, Churchill Livingstone. **B.** Courtesy Michael S. Clement, MD, Mesa, AZ.)

with the stethoscope and fetoscope. The *Doppler ultrasound* device transmits ultra-high-frequency sound waves to the moving interface of the fetal heart valves and deflects these back to the device, converting them into an electronic signal that can be counted. In addition, auscultation is useful to establish the point of maximum intensity of the fetal heart rate before initiating electronic fetal monitoring (to assist with placement of the external Doppler transducer), and to differentiate fetal heart rate from maternal heart rate.

Procedure	Rationale
1. Perform Leopold's maneuvers (Figure 3-2) by palpating the maternal abdomen.	1. To identify fetal presentation and position
2. Apply ultrasound gel to device if using a Doppler US. Place the listening device over the PMI (usually over the back of the fetus). If using the fetoscope, firm pressure may be needed.	2. To obtain the clearest and loudest sound (easier to count)
3. Count the maternal radial pulse.	3. To differentiate it from the fetal rate
4. Palpate the abdomen for the presence or absence of UA.	4. To be able to count the FHR between contractions
5. Count the FHR for 30 or 60 seconds between contractions.	5. To identify the auscultated rate (best assessed in the absence of UA)
6. Auscultate the FHR before, during, and after a contraction.	6. To identify the FHR during the contraction, as a response to the contraction, and to assess for the absence or presence of increases or decreases in FHR
7. When there are distinct discrepancies in fetal heart rate during listening periods, auscultate for a longer period during, after, and between contractions.	7. To identify significant changes that may indicate the need for another mode of FHR monitoring

Leopold's Maneuvers

Ensure the woman's bladder is empty.

Position woman supine with one pillow under her head and with her knees slightly flexed.

Place small rolled towel under her right hip to displace uterus (prevents supine hypotensive syndrome).

If right-handed, stand on woman's right, facing her:

1. Identify fetal part that occupies the fundus. The head feels round, firm, freely movable, and palpable by ballottement; the breech feels less regular and softer (identifies fetal lie [longitudinal or transverse] and presentation [cephalic or breech]; see Figure 3-2 A).

2. Using palmar surface of one hand, locate and palpate the smooth convex contour of the fetal back and the irregularities

that identify the small parts (feet, hands, elbows). This assists in identifying fetal presentation (see Figure 3-2 B).

3. With the right hand, determine which fetal part is presenting over the inlet to the true pelvis. Gently grasp the lower pole of the uterus between the thumb and fingers, pressing in slightly (see Figure 3-2 C below). If the head is presenting and not engaged, determine the attitude of the head (flexed or extended).

4. Turn to face the woman's feet. Using both hands, outline the fetal head (see Figure 3-2 D below) with palmar surface of fingertips. When presenting part has descended deeply, only a small portion of it may be outlined.

Palpation of cephalic prominence assists in identifying attitude of head.

If the cephalic prominence is found on the same side as the small parts, the head must be flexed, and the vertex is presenting. If

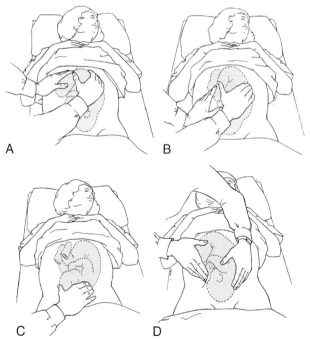

A

B

C

D

FIGURE 3-2 Leopold's maneuvers and determination of the PMI of the FHR. (From Lowdermilk DL, Perry SE: *Maternity & women's health care,* ed 9, St Louis, 2007, Mosby.)

the cephalic prominence is on the same side as the back, the presenting head is extended and the face is presenting.

To determine the point of maximal intensity of the fetal heart rate, see Box 3-1.

Frequency of Auscultation

Many countries prefer intermittent auscultation to continuous electronic fetal monitoring in women without risk factors, as this promotes their mobility, is less distracting, and provides a more natural birthing experience without the use of electronic devices. Reliance on the electronic monitor is more prevalent in the United States, most likely because of staffing patterns, staffing mix, and the increased use of defensive practices in a litigious environment. Regardless of the method used to assess the fetal heart rate, the standard practice is to evaluate and record the heart rate at specific intervals.

BOX 3-1   Determination of Point of Maximal Intensity of the Fetal Heart Rate

---

Perform Leopold's maneuvers.

Auscultate FHR on basis of fetal presentation. The PMI is the location where the FHR is heard the loudest, usually over the fetal back.

Determine fetal presentation, position, and lie; whether presenting part is flexed or extended, engaged or free floating.

Identify PMI of FHR using a two-line figure to indicate the four quadrants of the maternal abdomen, right upper quadrant (RUQ), left upper quadrant (LUQ), left lower quadrant (LLQ), and right lower quadrant (RLQ):

RUQ	LUQ
RLQ	LLQ

The umbilicus is the reference point for the quadrants (the point where the lines cross). The PMI for the fetus in vertex presentation, in general flexion with the back on the mother's right side, is commonly found in the mother's right lower quadrant and is recorded with an "X" or with the FHR as follows:

The American College of Obstetricians and Gynecologists[2] specifically states that "auscultation may not be appropriate for all pregnancies" and suggests continuous monitoring for patients with high-risk conditions. The American College of Nurse-Midwives[1] reviewed references from the United States, Canada, and Great Britain regarding the frequency of auscultation for low-risk women and found consistent recommendations for auscultation frequency of every 15 minutes in the active phase of the first stage of labor and every 5 minutes in the second stage. It is preferable to auscultate the fetal heart rate for at least 30 to 60 seconds. Nursing guidelines regarding the length and specific timing of auscultation are discussed in detail by the Association of Women's Health, Obstetric and Neonatal Nurses (AWHONN).[4]

Documentation of Auscultated Fetal Heart Rate

Documentation of the auscultated fetal heart rate must be accompanied by other routine parameters that are assessed during labor, including uterine activity, maternal observations and assessment, and both maternal and fetal responses to interventions. It should be noted how long the fetal heart rate was auscultated and whether this was before, during, and/or immediately after a uterine contraction. The rate, rhythm, and abrupt or gradual increases or decreases of the fetal heart rate during any part of this auscultated period should be described in relationship to uterine activity.

NOTE: It is *not* appropriate to describe auscultated fetal heart rate using the descriptive terms associated with electronic fetal monitoring because the majority of the electronic fetal monitoring terms are *visual descriptions* of the patterns produced on the monitor tracing (e.g., early, late, and variable decelerations or variability). However, terms that are numerically defined, such as bradycardia and tachycardia, can be used.

Interpretation of Auscultated Fetal Heart Rate

Reassuring Fetal Heart Rate

- FHR with a normal baseline range of 110 to 160 beats per minute (bpm)
- Regular rhythm (obtained between contractions), without wide fluctuations from the average rate

- Presence of increases from the baseline rate
- Absence of decreases from the baseline rate, assessed over a 10-minute period

Nonreassuring Fetal Heart Rate

- A baseline FHR of <110 bpm or >160 bpm
- Decreases in baseline FHR, with or without UA
- Irregular rhythm
- Decreased FHR from baseline, during and/or within 30 seconds after contractions

Management Options of a Nonreassuring Fetal Heart Rate

- Increase frequency of auscultation.
- Apply EFM to visualize pattern suspected or to assess baseline variability.
- Provide intrauterine resuscitation as appropriate.
- Perform vibroacoustic or scalp stimulation with electronic fetal monitoring to assess fetal response.

If a nonreassuring fetal heart rate persists after attempts to correct it, or if ancillary tests are not appropriate, then an expeditious delivery may be considered by the health care team.

Benefits and Limitations of Auscultation

Benefits

- Widely available and easy to use
- Less invasive
- Outcomes comparable to EFM with 1:1 nursing care
- Inexpensive
- Comfortable for the woman
- Provides freedom of movement for the woman
- Increases hands-on contact with the woman
- Allows easy FHR assessment during use of hydrotherapy

Limitations

- May be difficult to obtain the FHR in some situations, such as hydramnios and maternal obesity
- Does not provide a permanent, documented visual record of the FHR
- The counting of the FHR is intermittent
- Cannot assess visual patterns of the FHR variability or periodic changes

- Significant events may occur during periods when the FHR is not auscultated
- May not allow early detection of the fetal heart rate changes that reflect hypoxemia
- Not recommended for high-risk pregnancies

In summary, auscultation has been found to be effective if performed in a consistent manner by a clinician caring for a woman according to the prescribed frequency. Worldwide, auscultation is frequently and successfully employed as the first line of fetal assessment in low-risk populations. Continued research regarding auscultation, especially research related to nurse/patient ratios and frequency of assessments in latent phase labor, could prove beneficial in the acceptance of auscultation in the United States.

ELECTRONIC FETAL MONITORING

Overview

There are two modes of electronic monitoring. The external, or indirect, mode employs the use of external transducers placed on the maternal abdomen to assess the fetal heart rate and uterine activity. The internal, or direct, mode uses a spiral electrode (to assess the fetal heart rate) and an intrauterine pressure catheter (to assess uterine activity and intrauterine pressure) (Figures 3-3 and 3-4). In some countries, electronic fetal monitoring is called a cardiotocography or "CTG". The following chart compares the external and internal modes of monitoring and gives a brief description of the equipment used for each.

External Mode (Indirect)	Internal Mode (Direct)
Fetal Heart Rate	
US (Doppler) transducer: High-frequency sound waves reflect mechanical action of fetal heart.	**Spiral electrode:** Electrode converts fetal electrocardiogram (FECG) (as obtained from presenting part) to the fetal heart rate via cardiotachometer by measuring consecutive fetal R-wave intervals. The cervix must be sufficiently dilated to allow placement. The electrode penetrates the fetal presenting part 1.5 mm, and it must be securely attached to ensure an adequate signal.

External Mode (Indirect)	Internal Mode (Direct)

Uterine Activity

Tocodynamometer (tocotransducer): This instrument monitors the approximate frequency and duration of contractions by means of a pressure-sensing device applied to the abdomen.

Intrauterine catheter: This instrument monitors frequency, duration, and intensity of contractions and resting tone. The catheter is compressed during contractions, placing pressure on a transducer tip or the strain gauge mechanism of a fluid-filled catheter and then converting the pressure into millimeters of mercury (mm Hg) on the UA panel of the monitor tracing. The membranes must be ruptured and the cervix sufficiently dilated for placement. Catheters are available with a second lumen that can be used for amnioinfusion.

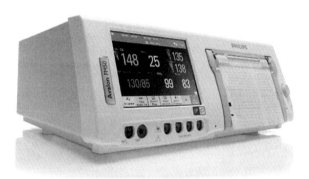

FIGURE 3-3 The Avalon 50 Fetal Monitor provides measurement of the FHR including noninvasive triplet monitoring, FHR high/low audible and visual alarms, and FECG. Maternal parameters include toco and intrauterine pressure, blood pressure, pulse rate, pulse oximetry, and ECG. It has cross-channel verification of maternal and fetal heart rate, displays FECG and MECG on the color-display touch screen, and integrates with the Avalon cordless transducer system. It is compatible with the OB TraceVue information management system and has a LAN interface for compatibility with hospital IT networks. (Courtesy Philips Medical Systems, Böblingen, Germany.)

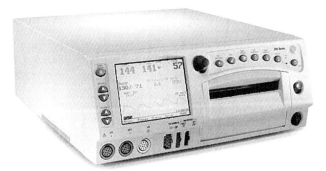

FIGURE 3-4 The Corometrics 250CX maternal/fetal monitor provides measurement of FHR, maternal UA, fetal movement detection, maternal blood pressure, pulse oximetry, and heart rate/ECG. It has FHR high/low alarms with audible and visual alerts and is compatible with Centricity Perinatal and other clinical information systems. (Courtesy GE Medical Systems Information Technologies, Milwaukee, WI.)

Converting Raw Data Into a Visual Display

The fetal heart rate and uterine activity data collected, whether by external or internal means, must then be converted into a visual display. This display may be on paper, a computer screen, or often both. Interpretation of electronic fetal heart rate monitoring is based on a visual assessment of data presented on a Cartesian graph. The gridlines on the horizontal (x) axis of the graph represent time in increments of 10 seconds. The gridlines on the vertical (y) axis represent the fetal heart rate in increments of 10 beats per minute. As illustrated in Figure 3-5, the fetal heart rate appears on the graph as an irregular horizontal line representing the fetal heart rate over a period of time. However, as demonstrated in Figure 3-6, closer inspection reveals that the "irregular horizontal line" is not a line at all. Instead, it is a series of individual, closely spaced points. Each point represents an individual heart rate that is calculated from the time between two successive heartbeats. This is a fundamental principle of electronic fetal heart rate monitoring and merits brief review.

Fetal monitoring equipment used in clinical practice detects the fetal heartbeat in one of two ways. A fetal scalp electrode detects the actual electrical impulses that originate in the fetal heart and make up the fetal electrocardiogram. An external transducer uses

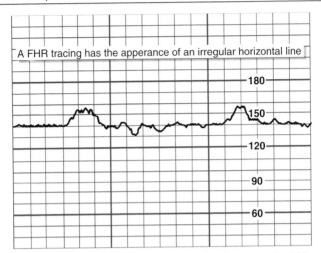

FIGURE 3-5 An FHR tracing has the appearance of an irregular horizontal line. (Courtesy David A. Miller, MD.)

Doppler ultrasound to detect cardiac motion. Regardless of the method of detecting the fetal heartbeat, the fetal heart rate monitor uses the same basic principles to process the raw data for visual display. If the fetal heart rate is derived from a direct fetal electrode detecting the fetal electrocardiogram, as illustrated in Figure 3-6,

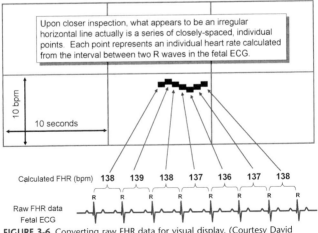

FIGURE 3-6 Converting raw FHR data for visual display. (Courtesy David A. Miller, MD.)

the monitor measures the distance between two successive R waves and calculates a heart rate based on that single R–R interval. The individual heart rate is plotted as a single point on the fetal heart rate graph. The monitor then measures the next R-R interval, calculates a new heart rate, and plots it as a new point on the graph. This process is repeated with every subsequent R wave. If the fetal heart rate is derived from an external Doppler ultrasound transducer, the monitor uses the peak of the Doppler waveform in place of the R wave and performs the same basic calculations. A normal fetal heart rate baseline rate of 140 beats per minute will yield approximately 140 individual graph points every minute, each representing an individual heart rate. To the eye, these individual points are spaced so closely together that they appear as a line. Variations in the fetal heart rate cause the line to appear irregular. The physiologic significance of these variations will be discussed in Chapter 5.

EXTERNAL MODE OF MONITORING

Ultrasound Transducer

Description

An ultrasound transducer is a device that is placed on the maternal abdomen and generates high-frequency ultrasound waves that are transmitted into the tissues (Figure 3-7). As the ultrasound waves strike tissue interfaces, some of the waves are reflected back toward the transducer from which they originated. The transducer detects the returning waves and converts them into electric signals. When ultrasound waves are reflected from a moving interface, such as the fetal heart, the waves return at different frequencies. This phenomenon is known as the Doppler effect. The change in frequencies can be used to calculate the motion of the target. As described previously, Doppler-detected fetal heart motion is converted to a continuous graphic display of fetal heart rate printed on the upper portion of the fetal heart rate monitor strip. Simultaneously, the Doppler-detected fetal heart rate is converted electronically to an audible beep and flashing light on the monitor. This Doppler signal can be affected by changes in the position of the transducer or the fetus. Changes in the direction of the sound beam during contractions may cause a loss of signal and make the resulting tracing uninterpretable.

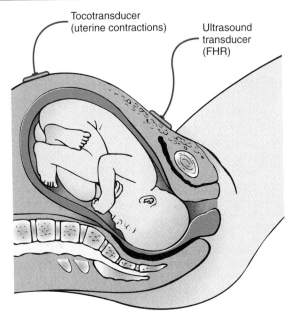

FIGURE 3-7 Placement of external transducers. The tocotransducer transmits UA. The US transducer transmits FHR. (From Lowdermilk DL, Perry SE: *Maternity & women's health care,* ed 9, St Louis, 2007, Mosby.)

Many monitors have dual ultrasound channels for the simultaneous monitoring of multiple fetuses. The two readings may be offset so that each fetal heart rate can more easily be identified (Figure 3-8).

The ultrasound transducer can be used to monitor the fetal heart rate during both antepartum and intrapartum periods. Correct placement of the ultrasound transducer depends on maternal cooperation and operator skill, because the transducer must usually be repositioned when the maternal position changes. Artifacts and erratic tracings may result from a number of causes, such as increased variability, halving or doubling of the fetal heart rate by the monitor, recording of maternal heart rate, fetal arrhythmias, and fetal or maternal movement.

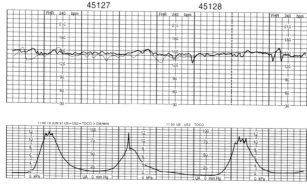

FIGURE 3-8 Dual US heart rate monitoring strip demonstrates the simultaneous external monitoring of twins. (Courtesy GE Medical Systems Information Technologies, Milwaukee, WI.)

Placement of Ultrasound Transducer

A sequential procedure with rationales is provided for the application of the ultrasound transducer.

Procedure	Rationale
1. Position the woman in a comfortable sitting or side-lying position.	1. To maximize uteroplacental blood flow by avoiding supine hypotension syndrome
2. Perform Leopold's maneuvers (see Figure 3-2).	2. To determine fetal position, lie, and presentation
3. Align and insert the US transducer plug into the appropriate monitor port (labeled cardio, or US for ultrasound).	3. To provide connection without damaging connector pins (could result in a faulty signal)
4. Apply US gel to the underside of the transducer placed on the maternal abdomen.	4. To aid in the transmission of US waves
5. Place the transducer on the abdomen, preferably over the fetal back, which is usually the PMI.	5. To achieve the clearest signal
6. Adjust the audio-volume control while moving the transducer over the abdomen.	6. To obtain the loudest audible fetal signal

Procedure	Rationale
7. Count the maternal radial pulse and compare with FHR.	7. To differentiate between maternal and fetal heart rates
8. Secure the US transducer with the abdominal belt or other fixation device.	8. To prevent displacement of the transducer
9. Observe the signal-quality indicator.	9. To verify clarity of input based on correct placement of the transducer
10. Set the recorder at a paper speed of 3 cm/min and observe the FHR on the monitor strip. NOTE: A speed of 1 or 2 cm/min is used in some countries.	10. To ensure that the paper feeds correctly and that the recording is clear
11. Reposition the transducer whenever the fetal signal becomes unclear (e.g., when the woman moves or when the fetus descends in the pelvis).	11. To ensure a clear, interpretable tracing during fetal monitoring
12. Carefully remove the transducer from the fixation device at the completion of monitoring, and cleanse the abdomen of gel.	12. To avoid damage to the transducer and to remove accumulated gel from the abdomen
13. Box 3-2 gives guidelines for care, cleaning, and storage of external transducers.	13. To prevent damage and ensure cleanliness of equipment

Tocotransducer

Description

The tocotransducer (toco) monitors uterine activity transabdominally by means of a pressure-sensing button that is depressed by uterine contractions or fetal movement. The uterine activity panel of the monitor paper displays the frequency and duration of contractions. Intensity and resting tone can be assessed only with palpation or the use of an intrauterine catheter. Thus, palpation of contractions to assess strength is mandatory when using the tocotransducer. The tocotransducer can be used to monitor uterine activity during both antepartum and intrapartum periods.

BOX 3-2   General Guidelines for Care, Cleaning, and Storage of External Transducers

- Exercise caution when removing and handling the US and tocotransducers so that they are not dropped or allowed to swing against any equipment, to protect from damage.
- Clean transducers according to the manufacturer's operating manual, usually with a soft cloth using mild soap and water. Avoid submerging transducers or placing them beneath running water. Do not use alcohol or other cleaning solutions that may damage equipment.
- Gently and loosely coil cables for storage. Avoid tight coiling and sharp bending of the cables, which will result in damage to the wires or casing.
- Cables between monitor models and manufacturers are usually not interchangeable. Forced insertion into an incompatible monitor port is likely to result in damage.
- Dispose of disposable abdominal belts. Wash reusable belts according to the facility's or the manufacturer's suggested procedure before the next use.

Placement of Tocotransducer

A sequential procedure with rationales is provided for the placement of the tocotransducer.

Procedure	Rationale
1. Gather the necessary equipment: fetal monitor, tocotransducer, and the equipment desired to monitor the FHR.	1. To ensure that all equipment is readily accessible
2. Position the woman in a comfortable semi-lateral position.	2. To maximize uteroplacental blood flow by avoiding supine hypotension syndrome
3. Perform Leopold's maneuvers (see Figure 3-2).	3. To determine fetal position, lie, and presentation
4. Align and insert the tocotransducer plug into the appropriate monitor port labeled Toco or UA.	4. To provide connection without damaging connector pins (could result in a faulty signal)
5. Place the transducer on the maternal abdomen over the upper uterine segment where there is the least amount of maternal tissue between the pressure-sensing button and the uterus (where uterine contractions are best palpated).	5. To ensure that the upper uterine segment is as close as possible to the pressure-sensing button

Procedure	Rationale
6. Secure the tocotransducer with the abdominal belt and ensure that there is no gel under the tocotransducer.	6. To prevent displacement of the transducer and to ensure that there is no gel accumulation that might impede function
7. Set the recorder at a paper speed of 3 cm/min, check the printed time/date for accuracy, and observe the monitor strip or computer screen. NOTE: A speed of 1 to 2 cm/min is used in some countries.	7. To ensure that the paper feeds correctly, the date is accurate, and the recording is clear and received by the monitoring system
8. Between contractions, press the UA or Toco test button for the resting baseline to print at the 20 mm Hg line on the monitor strip.	8. To prevent missing the very beginning or ending of the uterine contraction (necessary for the fetal heart rate pattern interpretation)
9. Monitor the frequency and duration of the contractions, and palpate the strength of the contractions as well as resting tone. Document them in the woman's medical record according to facility policy.	9. The tocotransducer *cannot* measure intensity of contractions or resting tone between contractions because the depression of the pressure-sensing button varies with amount of maternal adipose tissue; therefore the information should *not* be relied on to assess need for analgesia in relation to perceived strength (painfulness) of contractions as registered by the monitor
10. When monitoring is in progress, readjust abdominal belt periodically, and massage any reddened skin areas.	10. To promote comfort and maintain the proper position of the transducer
11. Reposition the transducer periodically and secure the abdominal belt snugly.	11. To promote and ensure a good recording
12. Carefully remove the transducer from the fixation device at the completion of monitoring.	12. To avoid damage to the transducer
13. See Box 3-2 for guidelines for care, cleaning, and storage of external transducers.	13. To prevent damage and ensure cleanliness of equipment

Advantages and Limitations of External Transducers

Advantages

- Noninvasive
- Easy to apply
- May be used during the antepartum period
- May be used with telemetry
- Does not require ruptured membranes or cervical dilation
- No known hazards to woman or fetus
- Provides continuous recording of the fetal heart rate and uterine activity

Limitations

- May limit maternal movement.
- Frequent repositioning of transducers is often needed to maintain an accurate tracing.
- US transducer (Doppler) may double-count a slow fetal heart rate of less than 60 bpm, resulting in an apparently normal fetal heart rate during a bradycardia; or it may half-count an elevated fetal heart rate of more than 180 bpm, resulting in an apparently normal fetal heart rate during a tachycardia.
- Maternal heart rate may be counted if the ultrasound transducer is placed over the maternal arterial vessels, such as the aorta.
- Tocotransducer provides information limited to frequency and duration of contractions; it cannot accurately assess strength or intensity of contractions.
- Obese women may be difficult to monitor.

INTERNAL MODE OF MONITORING

Spiral Electrode

Description

The spiral electrode monitors the fetal electrocardiogram from the presenting part. It is generally applied only after the membranes have been ruptured, although it may be applied through intact membranes when necessary.[3] Additionally, the cervix must be sufficiently dilated to allow placement and the presenting part must be accessible and identifiable (Figure 3-9). Therefore the spiral electrode is used only during the intrapartum period.

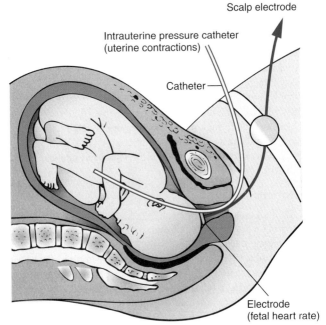

Scalp electrode

Intrauterine pressure catheter
(uterine contractions)

Catheter

Electrode
(fetal heart rate)

FIGURE 3-9 Diagrammatic representation of internal mode of monitoring with intrauterine pressure catheter and spiral electrode attached to fetal scalp. (From Lowdermilk DL, Perry SE: *Maternity & women's health care*, ed 9, St Louis, 2007, Mosby.)

Contraindications

- Planned application to the fetal face, fontanels, or genitalia
- Inability to identify the portion of the fetus where application is contemplated
- Presence or suspicion of placenta previa
- Presence of active herpes lesions or human immunodeficiency virus
- Maternal infection with hepatitis B or C

Situations Requiring Caution

- Woman is positive for group B streptococcus, syphilis, or gonorrhea
- The premature fetus

It is important to refer to the manufacturer's directions and guidelines, as well as current professional guidelines and institutional policies.

Placement of Fetal Spiral Electrode

A sequential procedure with rationales is provided for insertion and use of the spiral electrode.

Procedure	Rationale
1. Turn power on and insert cable into appropriate monitor port, labeled Cardio or ECG.	1. To connect cable plug to the appropriate outlet
2a. Apply gloves and perform a sterile vaginal examination to determine presenting fetal part.	2a. To maintain aseptic technique and to avoid the fetal face, fontanels, and genitalia
b. Retract spiral electrode until tip is approximately 1 inch into drive handle and introduce into vagina with non-examining hand, keeping examining fingers on target area.	b. To prevent damage to the vaginal wall, glove puncture, and injury to examining fingers during placement
c. Place the guide tube between the examining fingers and place firmly against the target area of the fetus.	c. To ensure proper placement
d. Rotate the drive and guide tubes *clockwise* approximately 1½ rotations until resistance is met. Do not continue to rotate the device.	d. To ensure proper depth of placement, and to avoid tissue injury from excessive placement depth
e. Release the electrode wires from the locking device or handle notch and slide the drive and guide tubes off the electrode wires and out of the vagina.	e. To maintain proper placement and safe removal of device
3. Discard the outer drive tube when the application procedure is completed.	3. To avoid contamination/exposure to blood and body fluids
4. Connect to the leg plate cable and secure on the woman's thigh.	4. To avoid tension, pulling, or dislodging the spiral electrode. The electrode must be securely attached to ensure a good signal.
5. Observe the signal-quality indicator.	5. To verify clear signal from electrode

Procedure	**Rationale**
6. Set the recorder at a paper speed of 3 cm/min, and observe the fetal heart rate on the strip chart. Note: A paper speed of 1 to 2 cm/min is used in some countries.	6. To ensure that the paper feeds correctly and that the recording is clear
7. During monitoring, check the attachment plate periodically, and reposition for comfort as needed.	7. To ensure transmission of the signal
8. When removing the spiral electrode, turn 1½ rotations *counter-clockwise* or until it is free from the fetal presenting part. Do not pull the electrode from the fetal skin. Do not cut wires and pull apart to remove electrode from the fetus. Disconnect the electrode from the leg plate, remove the attachment pad, and dispose of the electrode and the attachment pad according to facility policy.	8. To ensure that the electrode is removed in the same manner that it was applied; pulling the electrode straight out results in unnecessary trauma to the fetal skin, produces an observable wound, and predisposes the site to infection
9. The electrode should be removed just before cesarean delivery, vacuum extractor use, and forceps.	9. In cesarean delivery, the electrode should not be left attached and brought up through the uterine incision. If unable to detach, cut wire at perineum and notify physician.
10. Clean the leg plate cable, if reusable, according to the facility's procedure, or follow the directions in the manufacturer's operating manual.	10. To prevent infection
11. Loosely coil the cable and place in a secure area.	11. To prevent damage to the wires (can occur with tight coiling, resulting in loss of or an inadequate fetal signal)

Intrauterine Pressure Catheter

Description

The intrauterine pressure catheter or transducer (IUPC) monitors contraction frequency, duration, intensity, and resting tone (Figure 3-10). A small catheter is introduced through the vagina transcervically into the uterus after the fetal membranes have been ruptured and the cervix is sufficiently dilated to identify the presenting part. The catheter is compressed during uterine contractions, placing pressure on a transducer. The pressure is then reflected on the monitor tracing in units of millimeters of mercury (mm Hg).

Intrauterine pressure catheters that have the pressure-sensing device within the catheter tip or cable do not require an instillation of sterile water for use. These catheters are provided with an amnioport to allow simultaneous amniofusion while monitoring uterine activity. Always refer to the manufacturer's directions and guidelines, along with the facility's policies and procedures, for information on use and insertion.

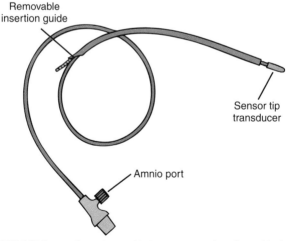

FIGURE 3-10 Intrauterine catheter with the sensor transducer located in the tip of the catheter provides uninterrupted UA monitoring. Saline-filled catheters are another type of catheter in use. Note that this catheter has an amnioport that may be used for an amnioinfusion.

Placement of Intrauterine Pressure Catheter

A licensed registered nurse may insert the intrauterine pressure catheter, but only if this is allowed by licensing board regulations and if the nurse is credentialed and approved by the institution's policies. The following chart shows the procedure in a sequential format for the use and insertion of the intrauterine pressure catheter.

Procedure	Rationale
1. Turn the power on and insert the reusable cable into the appropriate monitor connector labeled UA, Toco, or Utero.	1. To activate the pressure transducer
2. Depending on the make of catheter, zero the monitor after connecting to the cable and prior to insertion. Refer to manufacturer's directions for zeroing instructions.	2. To establish a zero baseline for the catheter system based on normal atmospheric pressure
3. If inserting a fluid-filled catheter, fill the catheter with 5 ml sterile water, leaving the syringe attached to the catheter. Maintain sterility at the maternal end of the catheter.	3. To ensure that the catheter is patent and fluid-filled before insertion; to maintain aseptic technique
4a. Perform a sterile vaginal examination and identify the fetal presenting part.	4a. To maintain aseptic technique and to identify the optimal location for catheter insertion
b. Insert the sterile catheter and introducer guide inside the cervix between the examining fingers; do not extend introducer guide beyond fingertips.	b. The guide is made of a hard plastic that can cause trauma if inserted farther than necessary.
c. Advance only the catheter according to the insertion depth indicator or until the blue/black or stop mark on it reaches the vaginal introitus.*	c. To ensure that enough of the catheter is inside the uterus (approximately 30 to 45 cm)

*Remove catheter immediately in the event of *extraovular* placement outside of the amniotic fluid space (between the chorionic membrane and endometrial lining), as evidenced by blood in the catheter.

Procedure	Rationale
d. Separate and remove or slide the catheter introducer guide away from the introitus and remove; dispose of the guide appropriately.	d. To prevent the guide from sliding toward the introitus
5. Secure the catheter to the woman's leg.	5. To ensure the woman's mobility without fear of dislodging the catheter
6. Encourage the woman to cough, or briefly perform a Valsalva maneuver. Observe the graph during this time; a sharp spike should appear when the IUPC is properly positioned.	6. To confirm placement and functioning
7. Document baseline resting tone in the supine position with left lateral and right lateral tilt.	7. To obtain baseline information, as maternal position and IUPC position may alter measurements
8. Re-zero monitor if indicated during labor, according to manufacturer's directions.	8. To ensure that UA information is correct
9. Gently remove catheter after use and discard; store reusable cable for future use.	9. To ensure that disposable catheter is not reused

Fluid-Filled Catheters

When monitoring is in progress:

a. Flush the intrauterine catheter with sterile water every 2 hours or as necessary (the use of solutions other than sterile water can occlude and corrode the system).	a. To remove any vernix caseosa or air bubbles that may have entered the catheter and can invalidate the pressure reading
b. Check the proper functioning of the catheter when necessary by tapping the catheter, asking the woman to cough, or performing a brief Valsalva maneuver while observing the chart.	b. To ensure proper function and confirm accurate recording on the chart paper

Advantages and Limitations of Internal Monitoring

Advantages

- Capability of accurately displaying some fetal cardiac arrhythmias when linked to ECG recorder
- Accurately displays a FHR between 30 and 240 bpm

- Only truly accurate measure of all UA (e.g., frequency, duration, intensity, and resting tone)
- Allows for use of amnioinfusion
- Positional changes do not usually affect quality of FHR tracing (may affect IUPC accuracy)
- May be more comfortable than external transducer belt

Limitations

- Presenting part must be accessible and identifiable to place fetal scalp electrode
- Internal electrode may record maternal heart rate in presence of fetal demise
- May not get good ECG conduction when excessive fetal hair is present
- Requires (or will result in) rupture of membranes
- Cervix must be dilated sufficiently to allow placement
- Improper insertion can cause maternal or placental trauma
- May increase risk for infection

A fetal monitoring equipment checklist (Table 3-1) can be used to check for and ensure proper functioning of the equipment. The woman who is electronically monitored should be given an explanation of equipment operations to allay any anxiety. The care given to the electronically monitored woman is the same as that given to any woman during labor, with the additional consideration of those factors that relate directly to the monitor.

DISPLAY OF FETAL HEART RATE, UTERINE ACTIVITY, AND OTHER INFORMATION

The display on the front of the monitor shows the fetal heart rate and the uterine pressure, and it identifies the signal source for each. Additional monitor options include maternal noninvasive blood pressure, maternal heart rate, maternal pulse rate, maternal electrocardiogram in real time, gross fetal body movements, and ST analysis (when using STAN®). These parameters are also displayed on the front or face of the monitor.

Other data, in addition to the fetal heart rate and uterine activity, may be printed on the monitor strip. The time of day, date, and paper speed are usually printed every 10 minutes. The signal source is usually printed on every three or four pages of the tracing and with each change of parameter and mode of monitoring. Depending on the monitor's options, other maternal and fetal data may be printed on the tracing. The maternal heart rate and maternal electrocardiogram

TABLE 3-1 Fetal Monitoring Equipment Checklist

Name: _____	Evaluator: _____			
Date: _____				
Items to Be Checked		**Yes**	**No**	**Remarks**

Preparation of Monitor
1. Is the paper inserted correctly?
2. Is the paper speed set for 3 cm/min speed?
3. Are the transducer cables plugged securely into the appropriate port?
4. Was the monitor date/time verified (when using electronic documentation)?

Ultrasound (US) Transducer
1. Has US transmission gel been applied to the transducer?
2. Was the FHR tested and noted on the monitor strip?
3. Was the FHR compared to the maternal pulse and noted?
4. Does a signal light flash or an audible beep sound with each heartbeat?
5. Is the belt secure and snug but comfortable?

Tocotransducer
1. Is the tocotransducer firmly positioned where there is the least maternal tissue?
2. Has the tocotransducer been applied without gel or paste?
3. Was the UA reference depressed between contractions?
4. Is the belt secure and snug but comfortable?

Spiral Electrode
1. Is the spiral electrode attached to the presenting part of the fetus?
2. Is the connecter attached firmly to the electrode pad (on the leg plate or abdomen)?
3. Is the inner surface of the electrode pad pre-gelled or covered with electrode gel?
4. Is the electrode pad properly secured to the mother's leg or abdomen?

IUPC
1. Is the length line on the catheter visible at the introitus?
2. Is it noted on the monitor paper that a test or calibration was done?
3. Has the monitor been set to zero according to the manufacturer's directions?
4. Is the IUPC properly secured to the patient?
5. Is baseline resting tone of uterus documented?

can be trended on the upper (or heart rate) section of the monitor strip. Maternal noninvasive blood pressure can also be printed as whole numbers. The manufacturer's operating manual should be available and referred to for more information, especially when assessing women with risk factors who may have concurrent monitoring of multiple parameters.

Monitor Tracing Scale

The fetal heart rate and uterine activity are printed on scaled paper. (Figure 3-11) The fetal heart rate is printed on the upper section and the uterine activity on the lower section. Monitors are preset by their manufacturers for the countries in which they are used. Note the differences in the range and scale of the fetal heart rate and uterine activity sections, as well as in the paper/recorder speed, in Figure 3-12. The monitor strip in Figure 3-12, *A*, depicts the tracing paper that is used with monitors used in North America, with a speed of 3 cm/min. The monitor strip in Figure 3-12, *B*, depicts the tracing paper that is used in many countries outside North America, with a speed of 1 cm/min. It is imperative to use paper that is correctly scaled to match the monitor settings.

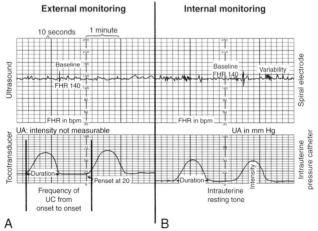

FIGURE 3-11 Display of FHR and UA on monitor strips. **A.** External mode of monitoring with US and toco as the signal source. **B.** Internal mode of monitoring with spiral electrode and intrauterine catheter as the signal source. Frequency of uterine contractions is measured from the onset of one contraction to the onset of the next.

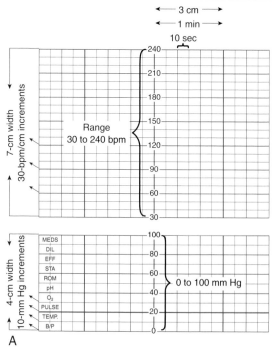

FIGURE 3-12 A. Fetal monitor paper scale: 3 cm/min speed used in North America.

Vertical Axis
Heart Rate
Range — 30 to 240 bpm
Scale — Increments of 30 bpm/cm
Uterine Activity
Range — 0 to 100 mm Hg pressure
Scale — Increments of 5 or 10 mm Hg
Horizontal Axis
Paper/recorder speed — 3 cm/min = six 10-second subsections within 1 minute

Continued

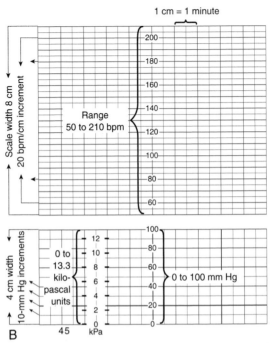

FIGURE 3-12, cont'd **B**. Fetal monitor paper scale: 1 cm per /min speed used in countries outside North America, with key points identified.

Vertical Axis
Heart Rate
Range   50 to 210 bpm
Scale   Increments of 20 bpm/cm
Uterine Activity
Range   0 to 100 mm Hg pressure, or 0 to
                           13.3 kilopascal units (1 kPa = 7.5 mm Hg)
Scale   Increments of 10 mm Hg
Horizontal Axis
Paper/recorder speed   1 cm/min = two subsections (or 2 cm/min
                           speed = four subsections)

Monitoring Twins and Multiples

Many monitors have the capability of monitoring twin or multiple gestations at the same time. Monitoring of twins may be done with two separate ultrasound transducers, or one fetus may be monitored by direct fetal scalp electrode (Figure 3-13). The dual tracings may be distinguished by a thicker or darker trace for one fetus and a thinner or lighter trace for the other fetus (see Figure 3-8). Another option to distinguish the tracings between twins is a "twin offset" mechanism, which separates the two fetal heart rates on the tracing by a distance of about 20 beats per minute. Thus one twin appears to have a fetal heart rate that is higher than the actual heart rate. The manufacturer's instruction manual should be consulted to have a clear understanding of this capability.

To clearly differentiate between twins, their positions in the uterus can be documented and ultrasound transducers labeled. The cross-channel verification alert may occur if both fetuses have the same/coincident heart rates. If this occurs, relocate the tocotransducer(s) to detect the second fetal heart rate. In identifying twins or multiples, the fetus in the advanced position just above the cervix is labeled A, the next one B, and so on.

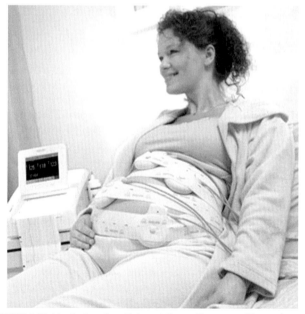

FIGURE 3-13 Monitoring of multiple gestations with separate US transducers. (Courtesy Philips Medical Systems, Böblingen, Germany.)

Artifact Detection

Fetal monitors have built-in artifact rejection systems, which are always in operation when using the external mode of fetal heart rate monitoring. Logic circuitry rejects data when there is a greater variation than is expected between successive fetal heartbeats. When repetitive variations vary by more than the accepted amount, newer monitors continue to print regardless of the extent of the excursion of the fetal heart rate.

The older generation of monitors may switch from a hold mode to a non-record mode. The recorder resumes recording when the variations between successive beats fall within the predetermined parameters.

During internal monitoring, artifact is rare, and the logic system will miss only those changes that exceed the predetermined limits of the system. If there is an accessible switch to select a logic or no-logic mode, it is preferable to have the monitor in the no-logic mode when using the internal mode (spiral electrode) to detect fetal arrhythmias. When recording internally, the logic-on mode should be used only when there is true artifact, such as when there is a low signal-to-noise ratio (caused by extraneous electrical noise), or when there is a large maternal R wave that is counted on an intermittent basis. This can usually be determined by printing out the fetal electrocardiogram.

Troubleshooting the Monitor

The electronic fetal monitor is a useful tool to assess fetal well-being. As with any electronic device, problems may occur, but they can often be overcome. A fetal monitoring equipment checklist (Table 3-1) can be used to screen for appropriate application of the monitor. The following chart suggests actions for identified electro-mechanical problems.

Problem	Action
Power	• Check power cord at wall and back of monitor.
Ultrasound	
Half or double rate	• Assess FHR with fetoscope, stethoscope, or Doppler.
	• Check maternal pulse to rule out maternal signal, and document maternal pulse.
	• Reapply US gel and recheck.
	• Move transducer to search for a better signal.
	• Consider applying spiral electrode.
Erratic trace or display	• Reposition transducer.
	• Reposition woman.
	• Tighten US belt if too loose.

Problem	Action
Erratic trace or display—cont'd	▪ Check gel on transducer (if it is dry, sound waves do not penetrate the skin). Reapply gel if needed. Move transducer if fetus is out of range.
Spiral Electrode	
Erratic trace or display	▪ Use a new spiral electrode. ▪ Check that reference electrode is in vaginal secretions (instill fluid if necessary). ▪ Check attachment pad on leg for adherence to skin. ▪ Ensure that connection of electrode is secure on attachment pad and that connector is securely inserted into the leg-plate cable.
Signal-quality indicator is continuously red	▪ Ensure that logic switch is off to assess for fetal arrhythmia.
Tocotransducer	
Not recording	▪ Check that cable is plugged into monitor and power is on.
Numbers in high range	▪ Readjust toco on abdomen; ensure that cable is fully attached to monitor. ▪ Zero monitor with toco/UA button between contractions, or replace with another toco.
Toco not picking up contractions	▪ Palpate abdomen for best location to sense contractions, and reapply toco. ▪ Test toco by depressing pressure transducer and observing readout on monitor. ▪ Tighten belt, or use another device to hold toco firmly against abdomen. ▪ Consider using IUPC.
Intrauterine Pressure Catheter	
Not recording	▪ Recheck cable insertion. ▪ Flush fluid-filled catheter.
Resting tone (>25 mm Hg)	▪ Palpate abdomen to identify uterine tonus before making equipment adjustments. ▪ Adjust level of strain gauge for fluid-filled catheters to maternal xyphoid. ▪ Zero or recalibrate non–fluid-filled catheter. ▪ Flush fluid-filled catheter.
Not recording contractions	▪ Check catheter markings at woman's introitus (catheter may have slipped out). ▪ Replace catheter if necessary.

Problem	Action
High resting tone	<ul><li>Higher resting tone may be noted with multiple gestation, uterine malformation or fibroids, use of oxytocin, amnioinfusion, extraovular placement.</li><li>Decrease or discontinue oxytocin or amnioinfusion in presence of uterine hypertonus</li><li>Re-zero monitor.</li><li>Replace catheter if incorrect placement.</li></ul>
Other Issues	
Fetal arrhythmia	Auscultate fetal heart rate with fetoscope or stethoscope.<ul><li>Check for tachycardia or bradycardia.</li><li>Perform FECG.</li></ul>
Errors caused by incorrect paper speed or paper with different scale	<ul><li>Check annotation with paper speed: it should be 3 cm/min in North America.</li><li>Check scale: it should be 30 to 240 bpm for fetal heart rate if paper speed is 3 cm/min, or 50 to 210 bpm if paper speed is 1 or 2 cm/min.</li></ul>
Cross-channel verification alert	<ul><li>Alert occurs with two coincidental heart rates. Verify maternal heart rate. Reposition US transducer(s) to detect second FHR.</li></ul>

Telemetry

Remote internal or external fetal heart rate monitoring via radio wave telemetry (Figure 3-14) helps women remain ambulatory without the loss of continuous monitoring data. A woman may feel less confined, more relaxed, and more content if she can walk around. The transducer is worn by means of an abdominal belt or other device (Figure 3-15). Heart rate and uterine activity signals are continuously transmitted to a receiver that is connected to the fetal monitor. The monitor then processes and displays the data, and it prints the heart rate and uterine activity on the monitor strip. Use of a central display facilitates clinician surveillance of the telemetry-monitored patient.

In addition to standard ultrasound and tocotransducers, external watertight transducers are available. These can be used to continue fetal surveillance during hydrotherapy or waterbirth. For example, a woman can use a watertight transducer with a wireless telemetry device when in a shower, spa, or tub.

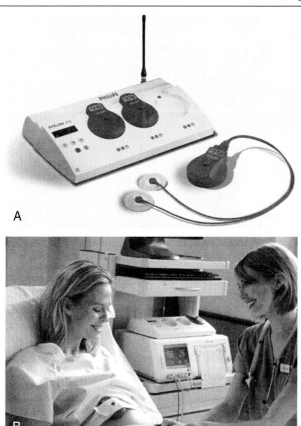

FIGURE 3-14 A. The cordless transducer system (Avalon CTS) combines fetal monitoring technology with radio frequency technology to transmit information to a base station. This system eliminates the need for cables. Waterproof transducers may be used for the patient who is in bed, ambulating, or in the bath. **B.** Cordless US and tocotransducers are applied to the maternal abdomen for external monitoring. The base station above the fetal monitor is compatible with Philips, HP, and Agilent Series 50 fetal monitors. An automated frequency search at the base station prevents confusion of transducers with multiple systems. (Courtesy Philips Medical Systems, Böblingen, Germany.)

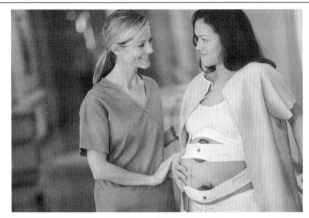

FIGURE 3-15 The cordless transducer system allows the woman mobility, providing a choice of positions while the fetus is being monitored. (Courtesy Philips Medical Systems, Böblingen, Germany.)

In addition to providing the benefits of freedom of movement during labor and continuous monitoring in the labor suite or the delivery room, telemetry has been applied in the outpatient setting for women instructed to remain at rest in their own homes. Data from the transmitter can be sent via modem to the receiver unit, which is connected to a printer, producing a hard copy of the fetal heart rate monitor strip. This transmission of information from the woman to the receiver unit allows the clinician to determine the woman's status. With the data received, the clinician can adjust the woman's care and can also consult with a referral center and receive an expert's interpretation of the data.

Central Displays

A central monitor display at the nurses' station provides an opportunity to view tracings from several women at the same time (Figure 3-16). Single-screen displays of several women or of one woman can be accessed from remote locations, including the bedside, the staff locker room or lounge area, the physician's office, or at home. Thus the staff can have instant access to the monitor patterns from many locations, which is especially important when a nurse cannot be in constant attendance. Some systems include the capability of data entry in the form of detailed notes about examination results, cervical dilation, fetal station, administration of drugs, the woman's position, and vital signs,

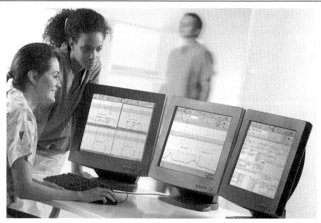

FIGURE 3-16 Central display for EFM allowing access to multiple records in a variety of formats. (Courtesy Philips Medical Systems, Böblingen, Germany.)

all related to time. Reports can even be generated with a printer linked to the display, which can provide a single and comprehensive document containing information, history, and a graphic printout of the labor curve progression.

Some central display systems can provide additional information (Figure 3-17), including the following:

- A *system status* screen provides an instant overview of several beds on the system and indicates any alerts by room number. In addition, it can identify the signal source of any woman on the system.
- A *trend screen* can provide the most recent few minutes of heart rate and UA data on any one woman, with immediate warning of critical conditions relating to any woman in the system.
- An *alert screen* can provide an immediate summary of the trend analysis on any woman. The data can be made available to the staff before, during, and after an alert.

Computer-Based Information Systems

Rapid advances in informatics technology have resulted in systems that combine fetal surveillance and alerting with documentation, data

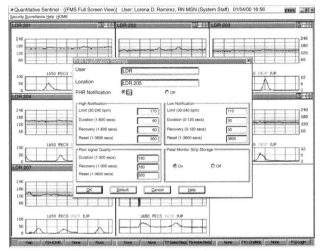

FIGURE 3-17 The surveillance system provides an overview of many women. It also allows the user to set the high/low ranges that will initiate an audible or visual notification of fetal bradycardia and tachycardia. If the heart rate violates the set limits and duration, the notification will continue until it has been acknowledged, even if the heart rate returns to an acceptable level. High/low ranges may be set at different levels for each woman. (Courtesy GE Medical Systems Information Technologies, Milwaukee, WI.)

storage, and retrieval. Such systems can cover the entire continuum of obstetric care across several pregnancies. The surveillance component of the system can be set to alert for fetal tachycardia or bradycardia, signal loss, coincidental fetal and maternal heart rates, and other parameters. Ranges for the duration of, and recovery from, fetal bradycardia or tachycardia can be set at different levels for each patient. These systems are widely available from a variety of companies.

In addition to improving the quality of care through surveillance and alert capabilities, a system that is accessible across the health care continuum can also provide a database for statistical reporting for administration, research, and quality purposes, especially when integrated with other hospital or outpatient information systems. Such a system can provide multiple data entry points across the continuum of care and on the various campuses of a hospital network.[5] These points include the physician's office, ambulatory care clinic, antepartum testing center, inpatient department, labor and delivery suite or birthing center, and home health or continuing care department. For example, if a woman presents to the birthing center in the middle of the night, the staff can readily access the entire antenatal record, the home uterine monitoring documents, and the ultrasound report, nonstress test, and biophysical profile that were completed just the previous afternoon, even at a different campus within the system. Additionally, some systems allow clinicians to access information and review fetal heart rate tracings using cellular phone displays (Figure 3-18).

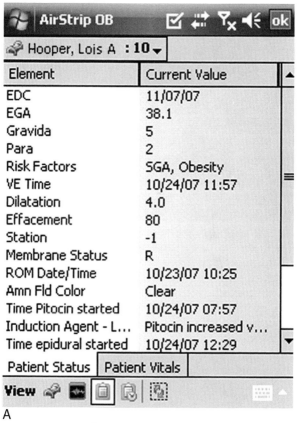

A

FIGURE 3-18 Airstrip OB® allows providers real-time remote access to patient data via a cellular connection. **A.** Overview of patient statistics. (Courtesy Airstrip Technologies, San Antonio, TX.)

Continued

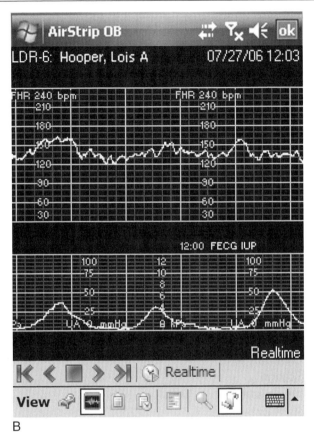

FIGURE 3-18 cont'd **B.** Real-time view of fetal monitor strip.

Documentation on forms and flow sheets, together with anno-
tated tracings, can quickly and easily provide complete electronic
patient records. The *archival* and *retrieval* of the original fetal monitoring strip has proved to be a problem for most medical record
departments because the process is labor intensive and the paper is
space consuming. Microfiche records are less bulky to store but still
take time to log, sort, and file in the medical record, although many
facilities continue to do this. A welcome alternative has been computer-based storage systems on the hard drive and optical laser
disks. These systems are best installed with a security system that

prevents alteration or removal of the documents, and a backup system in the event that there is damage or loss of the optical disk cartridge.

The ability to have multiple points of data entry, information retrieval, and reproduction of a woman's record and fetal monitor tracing is a significant advancement. This, coupled with an interface to the hospital admission, discharge, and transfer information system and other hospital-based information systems, should contribute to the trend toward comprehensive, paperless, and fully electronic information systems.

Data-Input Devices

Data-input devices can be used with electronic fetal monitors and monitoring systems. Some of their options include use of a bar-code reader, keypads for data entry, light-pens (Figure 3-19), touch screens, remote event markers, and standard keyboards. The input is subsequently printed on the tracing (Figure 3-20). The use of these options can promote accurate documentation and help eliminate the need for handwritten annotations, which are

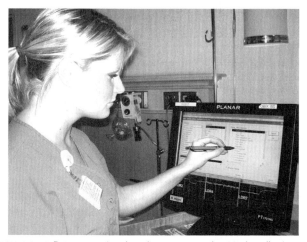

FIGURE 3-19 Data entry using drop-down menus and pen stylus, allowing nurse to chart directly using computer screen. (Courtesy OBiX Perinatal System, Clinical Computer Systems, Inc., Elgin, IL)

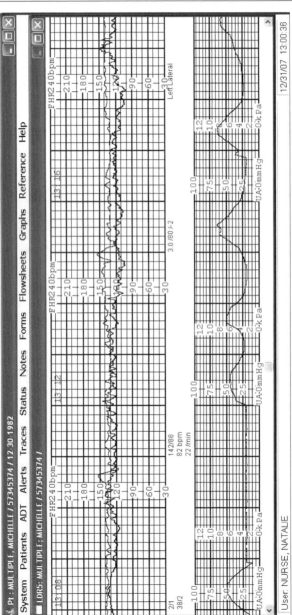

FIGURE 3-20 Sample tracing demonstrating display of patient data, including nursing assessments and interventions. Note FHR tracing of twins. (Courtesy OBiX Perinatal System, Clinical Computer Systems, Inc., Elgin, IL)

sometimes illegible. Additional information may be entered on the monitor strip automatically, such as the time, date, paper speed, and signal source. For more on documentation and electronic medical records, see Chapter 10, "Patient Safety, Risk Management, and Documentation."

ST Segment Analysis

As an adjunct to electronic fetal monitoring, clinicians may now access information regarding the ST segment of the fetal electrocardiogram during labor with an ST waveform analyzer (STAN®; Neoventa Medical, Göteborg, Sweden)[6] Using a combination of fetal heart rate interpretation guidelines and ST waveform analysis, STAN® provides clinicians with information on the fetal myocardial response to hypoxia based on fetal electrocardiogram changes, specifically changes in the ST interval.

The STAN® system consists of an electronic fetal monitoring monitor with a special ST analysis feature (Figure 3-21). The monitor can be used with or without ST analysis, functioning as a standard fetal monitor with all gestational ages; however, use of the adjunctive ST analysis option requires several patient characteristics be met:

- Planned vaginal delivery
- >36 completed weeks of gestation
- Singleton fetus
- Vertex presentation
- Ruptured amniotic membranes

Once appropriate patient selection has been determined, a special scalp electrode is applied (Figure 3-22) and fetal electrocardiogram data are analyzed to evaluate the T/QRS ratio and the ST interval (Figure 3-23). These data are evaluated and appear on the monitor screen below the electronic fetal monitoring tracing (Figure 3-24). Clinicians apply strict classification and analysis guidelines to determine the fetal response to hypoxia and subsequent labor management. Further information on STAN® as an adjunct to electronic fetal monitoring is presented in Chapter 6.

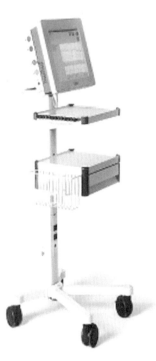

FIGURE 3-21 The STAN® S31 fetal monitor, capable of both traditional EFM and adjunctive ST waveform analysis for selected patients. (Courtesy Neoventa Medical, Mölndal, Sweden.)

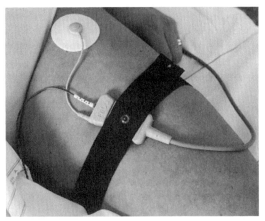

FIGURE 3-22 Applied spiral scalp electrode and skin electrode. (Courtesy Neoventa Medical, Mölndal, Sweden.)

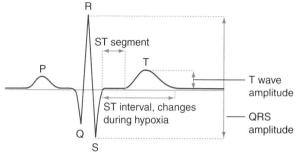

FIGURE 3-23 FECG complex illustrating the relationship of various parameters evaluated by STAN® (Courtesy Neoventa Medical, Mölndal, Sweden.)

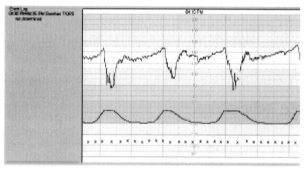

FIGURE 3-24 Computer screen showing EFM tracing (upper graph) with ST analysis data (lower graph). (Courtesy Neoventa Medical, Mölndal, Sweden.)

References

1. American College of Nurse-Midwives: Intermittent auscultation for intrapartum fetal heart rate surveillance. ACNM *Clinical Bulletin* no. 9, *J Nurse Midwifery* 52:314-319, 2007.

2. American College of Obstetricians and Gynecologists: Intrapartum fetal heart rate monitoring. ACOG *Practice Bulletin* no.70, *Obstet Gynecol* 106(6):1453-1461, 2005.

3. Association of Women's Health, Obstetric, and Neonatal Nurses (AWHONN) Amniotomy and Placement of Internal Fetal Spiral Electrode Through Intact Membranes: *Clinical Position Statement*, 2004.

4. Feinstein NF, Sprague A, Trépanier MJ: *Fetal heart rate auscultation*, Washington, DC, 2000, Association of Women's Health, Obstetric and Neonatal Nurses (AWHONN).

5. Kelly CS: Perinatal computerized patient record and archiving systems: Pitfalls and enhancements for implementing a successful computerized medical record. *J Perinat Neonatal Nurs* 12(4):1-14, 1999.
6. Rosen KG, Lindencrantz K: STAN—the Gothenburg model for fetal surveillance during labour by ST analysis of the fetal electrocardiogram. *Clin Phys Physiol Meas* 10(Suppl B):51-56, 1989.

Bibliography

American Academy of Pediatrics (AAP), American College of Obstetricians and Gynecologists (ACOG): *Guidelines for perinatal care*, ed 6, Washington, DC, 2007, AAP and ACOG.

Association of Women's Health, Obstetric and Neonatal Nurses (AWHONN): *Fetal heart monitoring: Principles and practices*, ed 3, Dubuque, Iowa, 2003, Kendall/Hunt.

Fraser DM, Cooper MA, editors: *Myles textbook for midwives*, ed 14, London, 2003, Churchill Livingstone.

Lowdermilk DL, Perry SE: *Maternity & women's health care*, ed 9, St Louis, 2007, Mosby.

Neoventa: *Fetal monitoring and ST analysis*, Chicago, 2007, Neoventa Medical, Inc.

Westerhuis M, Kwee A, van Ginkel A, Drogtrp A, Gyselaers W, Visser G: Limitations of ST analysis in clinical practice: Three cases of intrapartum metabolic acidosis. *BJOG,* DOI: 10.1111/j.1471-0528.2007.01236.

Evaluation of Uterine Activity

The primary objective of intrapartum fetal heart rate (FHR) monitoring is to prevent fetal injury that might result from disrupted fetal oxygenation during labor. Accurate assessment and management of uterine activity (UA) is crucial to achieving that goal. Excessive uterine activity can result in an interruption of fetal oxygenation and has been linked to an increased incidence of fetal acidemia of all types.[6,8,21] This chapter will focus on the evaluation of uterine activity in labor, including defining both normal and excessive uterine activity and the diagnosis and management of abnormal labor patterns. Additionally, specific issues regarding assessment of uterine activity associated with the use of oxytocin and risk management strategies related to uterine activity and labor stimulation are addressed.

ASSESSMENT METHODS: PALPATION AND ELECTRONIC MONITORING

Assessment of uterine activity includes the identification of contraction frequency, duration, strength or intensity, and resting tone. Uterine activity may be assessed by manual palpation or by electronic monitoring with either a tocotransducer or an internal intrauterine pressure catheter (IUPC). Differences in the accuracy of uterine activity evaluation are illustrated in Figure 4-1.

Palpation

Manual palpation is the traditional method of monitoring contractions. This method can measure contraction frequency, duration, and relative strength. Palpation is a learned skill that is best performed with the fingertips to feel the uterus rise upward as the contraction develops. *Mild, moderate,* and *strong* are the terms used to describe the strength of uterine contractions as determined by the examiner's hands during palpation and based on the degree of indentation of the abdomen.[5,18] For learning and for the purpose of comparison, the degree of indentation corresponds to the palpation

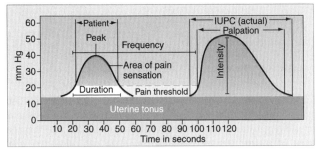

FIGURE 4-1 Comparison of relative sensitivities of assessing uterine contractions by internal monitoring (IUPC), manual palpation, and patient perception. Note that the woman does not usually perceive the contraction until the uterine pressure increases above the baseline. External monitor is variable. (Modified from Dickason EJ, Silverman BL, Kaplan JA: *Maternal-infant nursing care,* ed 3, St Louis, 1998, Mosby.)

sensation when feeling the parts of the adult face, as described in the following chart:

Contraction Strength	Palpation Sensation
Mild	Tense fundus but easy to indent (feels like touching finger to tip of nose)
Moderate	Firm fundus, difficult to indent with fingertips (feels like touching finger to chin)
Strong	Rigid, board-like fundus, almost impossible to indent (feels like touching finger to forehead)

The majority of labors in the world are managed by palpation, which promotes maternal ambulation and freedom of movement. Palpation as the sole method of monitoring uterine activity is less frequent in hospitals in North America than in other countries.

Electronic Monitoring

Electronic monitoring provides continuous data and a permanent record of uterine activity. *External uterine activity monitoring* is achieved using a tocotransducer (to provide information about uterine contraction frequency and duration) combined with manual palpation (to evaluate relative strength). The electronic display of a contraction depends on the depression of a pressure-sensing device placed on the maternal abdomen. Factors such as placement of the transducer, belt tightness, and maternal adipose tissue result in

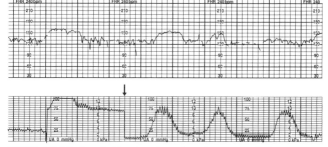

FIGURE 4-2 Adjustment of tocotransducer *(arrow)* to correct displacement following maternal position change. Note the tocotransducer picking up maternal breathing movements *(highlighted)*. (Courtesy Lisa A. Miller, CNM, JD.)

variations of depression and will affect the graphic representation on the fetal heart rate tracing (Figure 4-2). Thus the contractions may appear stronger (or less strong) than they truly are, making it imperative to assess strength of the uterine contraction by manual palpation when uterine activity is externally monitored.

Internal uterine activity monitoring uses an intrauterine pressure catheter that measures actual intrauterine pressure in millimeters of mercury (mm Hg) during both contractile and acontractile (resting) periods. As demonstrated in Figure 4-1, the intrauterine pressure catheter allows clinicians to evaluate the frequency, duration, and strength of contractions in mm Hg with improved accuracy. The following chart contrasts the data obtained with these two modes of monitoring:

External Mode - Tocotransducer	Internal Mode - Intrauterine Pressure Catheter
Frequency of Contractions	
Measured from the onset of one contraction to the onset of the next contraction	Measured from the onset of one contraction to the onset of the next contraction
Duration of Contractions	
Measured from contraction onset to offset	Measured from contraction onset to offset
Strength/Intensity of Contractions	
The abdomen must be palpated to assess the strength of the contraction based on the degree of indentation of the fundus. The more difficult it is to indent the fundus during palpation,	Intensity of contractions is measured directly and reflected on the tracing based on the intrauterine pressure in mm Hg. Intensity is recorded as the numerical value at the peak of

External Mode - Tocotransducer	Internal Mode - Intrauterine Pressure Catheter

Strength/Intensity of Contractions—Cont'd

the stronger the contraction. The tracing produced using a tocotransducer will reflect contraction strength *relative* to other contractions; i.e., stronger contractions will generally produce higher waveforms.

the contraction, e.g., 50 mm Hg, 70 mm Hg, etc. The tracing produced using an internal pressure catheter will reflect the *actual* intensity of the contractions, as expressed in mm Hg.

Resting Tone

The abdomen must be palpated to assess resting tone based on whether the fundus palpates as soft or firm (rigid). During periods of palpated resting tone the external monitor is generally set/reset to a level of 10 on the UA portion of the fetal monitoring tracing.

Resting tone is measured directly and reflected on the tracing based on the intrauterine pressure in mm Hg. Resting pressure is recorded as the numerical value when the uterus is completely relaxed (acontractile), e.g., 10 mm Hg, 15 mm Hg, etc.

Electronic Display of Uterine Activity

Uterine activity is monitored and recorded on the lower section of the monitor strip (Figure 4-3). The range of the scale is from 0 to 100 mm Hg. There are five major vertical divisions of 20 mm Hg each, divided again into minor vertical representations of 10 mm Hg each. Some tracing paper manufactured in North America has four major vertical sections of 25 mm Hg each, with the smaller divisions representing

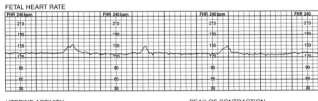

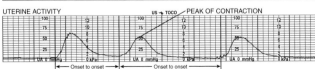

FIGURE 4-3 Frequency of uterine contractions can be measured from the onset of one UC to the onset of the next. Note other identifying information. (Courtesy Lisa A. Miller, CNM, JD.)

5 mm Hg pressure in the uterine activity section. For further information on instrumentation, please refer to Chapter 3.

STAGES OF NORMAL LABOR

The first stage of labor begins with the onset of contractions and ends with complete dilation of the cervix. It is divided into two phases: latent and active. During the latent phase, irregular and infrequent uterine contractions are associated with gradual cervical softening, dilation, and effacement (thinning). During the active phase of labor, the rate of cervical dilation increases and the fetal presenting part descends. The progress of labor can be plotted on a partogram or cervicograph, providing a visual record of cervical dilation and descent of the presenting part over time (Figure 4-4). As the fetal presenting part descends and cervical dilation increases, the lines cross each other in an **x** pattern. The progression of labor may be identified as normal, dysfunctional, or precipitous.

DEFINING NORMAL UTERINE ACTIVITY

Much of the data defining the "normal" range of uterine activity was derived from the research of Caldeyro-Barcia and colleagues[9-13] in the late 1950s and the 1960s. Using intra-amniotic pressure catheters, Caldeyro-Barcia and Poseiro[11] evaluated uterine activity and coined the term *Montevideo units (MVUs)* as a method of measuring uterine activity. The original formula was calculated by multiplying the average intensity in mm Hg (peak of contraction less baseline tone) times the frequency of uterine contractions in a 10-minute period. Thus, if there are 4 contractions in 10 minutes with an average intensity of 40 mm Hg, the Montevideo units for that period would be 4×40, or 160 Montevideo units. Over time, it became obvious that simple *addition* of the individual contraction intensities over 10 minutes resulted in essentially similar numbers to the multiplication method and since then the addition method has become common practice.[5]

Labor was found to begin clinically when Montevideo units rose to between 80 and 120, with contraction strength needing to reach at least 40 mm Hg.[10,11] This would equate to two to three contractions with intensities of 40 mm Hg or more every 10 minutes for the initiation of labor. In normal labor, contractions increase in intensity and frequency as labor progresses through the first stage and into the second stage. Caldeyro-Barcia and colleagues[10-12] found that

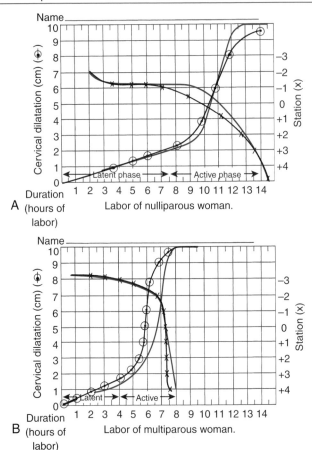

FIGURE 4-4 Partogram for assessment of patterns of cervical dilation and descent. Individual woman's labor patterns *(black)* superimposed on prepared labor graph for comparison. **A.** Labor of a nulliparous woman. **B.** Labor of a multiparous woman. The rate of cervical dilation is plotted with the circled plot points. A line drawn through these symbols depicts the slope of the curve. Station is plotted with Xs. A line drawn through the Xs reveals the pattern of descent. (Modified from Lowdermilk DL, Perry SE: *Maternity & women's health care,* ed 9, St Louis, 2007, Mosby.)

uterine activity in normal labor generally ranged between 100 and 250 Montevideo units, with contractions increasing in intensity from 25 to 50 mm Hg and in frequency from three to five over 10 minutes. It was also noted that the value of 250 Montevideo units was "very rarely surpassed in normal labor."[12] Baseline uterine tone averaged 10 mm Hg during labor, rising from 8 to 12 mm Hg from the beginning of the first stage to the onset of the second stage. In the second stage, Montevideo units can rise to 300 to 400,[6,9-13] as contraction intensities may increase to 80 mm Hg or more and five or six contractions may be seen every 10 minutes. Contraction duration of 60 to 80 seconds remains relatively stable from active phase labor through the second stage.[22] These findings provide a basis for logical definitions of "adequate" or "normal" uterine activity when using internal pressure catheters for assessment of uterine contractions.

Caldeyro-Barcia and Poseiro also provided crucial information related to contraction assessment when using palpation, or palpation and a tocotransducer. They found that until the intensity (peak less baseline tonus) reaches 40 mm Hg, the wall of the uterus is easily indented by palpation.[10] This correlates well with the premise that uterine contractions that palpate as moderate or stronger are likely to have peaks of 50 mm Hg or greater if they are measured by internal means, whereas palpated contractions identified as mild are likely to have peaks of less than 50 mm Hg if measured internally. These findings offer guidance for clinicians in identifying reasonable definitions of "adequate" or "normal" uterine activity when using palpation (with or without a tocotransducer) for assessment of uterine contractions. Box 4-1 provides a summary of normal uterine activity patterns in labor.

In summary, applying what is known about parameters of normal uterine activity:

1. allows clinicians to promote and support adequate and effective uterine activity during the different phases and stages of labor, influencing management decisions when abnormal or dysfunctional labor is diagnosed,
2. forms a basis for the safe and proper use of labor stimulants, and
3. provides a basis upon which to define excessive uterine activity by professional consensus.

DEFINING EXCESSIVE UTERINE ACTIVITY

Greater than normal uterine activity has long been linked to untoward effects on fetal heart rate tracings.[8,32] Peebles[21] noted decreased fetal cerebral oxygen saturation with shorter contraction intervals. Bakker and colleagues[6] found that fetal acidemia (umbilical artery pH ≤ 7.11) of all types (respiratory, metabolic, and mixed) was more

BOX 4-1   Normal Uterine Activity During Labor

Frequency	Contraction frequency overall generally ranges from 2 to 5 per 10 minutes during labor, with lower frequencies seen in the first stage of labor and higher frequencies (up to 6 contractions in 10 minutes) seen during the second stage of labor.
Duration	Contraction duration remains fairly stable throughout the first and second stages, ranging from 45 to 80 seconds, not generally exceeding 90 seconds.
Intensity (peak less resting tone)	Intensity of uterine contractions generally range from 25-50 mm Hg in the first stage of labor and may rise to over 80 mm Hg in second stage. Contractions palpated as "mild" would likely peak at less than 50 mm Hg if measured internally, whereas contractions palpated as "moderate" or greater would likely peak at 50 mm Hg or greater if measured internally.
Resting tone	Average resting tone during labor is 10 mm Hg; if using palpation, should palpate as "soft", i.e., easily indented, no palpable resistance.
MVUs	Ranges from 100 to 250 MVUs in the first stage, may rise to 300 to 400 in the second stage. Contraction intensities of 40 mm Hg or more and MVUs of 80 to 120 are generally sufficient to initiate spontaneous labor.

prevalent in patients with excessive uterine activity during labor, both first and second stage. Specifically, a first stage average Montevideo units value of 261 and a second stage average Montevideo units value of 442 was noted in the acidemic group, versus averages of 236 and 402 Montevideo units, respectively, in the first and second stages of the non-acidemic group.[6] Logic would therefore dictate that *avoiding* Montevideo unit values exceeding the previously discussed norm of 250 in the first stage of labor and 300 to 400 in the second stage could *decrease* the incidence of fetal acidemia at birth. Excessive uterine activity, especially in relation to oxytocin management, is one of the top sources of conflict between nurses and physicians.[34] Regrettably, professional guidelines concerning fetal monitoring, in both the United States and Europe, provide little information related to uterine activity.[6]

Compounding this issue is the lack of sound, standardized definitions for terms such as *hyperstimulation, hypertonus,* and *tachysystole*. Historically, the term *tachysystole* (from the Greek *tachy* meaning "rapid" and *systole* meaning "contraction") was used to describe excessive uterine activity. Introduction of the use of synthetic oxytocin to induce or augment (i.e., "stimulate") labor resulted in clinicians adopting the term *hyperstimulation* (*hyper* to reflect excessive, *stimulation* reflecting involvement of an external, or exogenous, stimulus). Over time, clinicians began to use the terms interchangeably, to reflect excessive uterine activity whether it was occurring spontaneously (*tachysystole*) or in response to labor stimulants (*hyperstimulation*).

Conflict regarding these definitions is a frequent occurrence among perinatal team members and a common concern raised at national fetal monitoring education programs. Even within organizations there appears to be conflict. The American College of Obstetricians and Gynecologists (ACOG) in one source directly defines *hyperstimulation* as "a persistent pattern of more than 5 contractions in 10 minutes, contractions lasting 2 minutes or more, or contractions of normal duration occurring within 1 minute of each other,"[2] while another ACOG source refers tangentially to both *hyperstimulation* and *hypertonus,* defining the terms parenthetically: "hyperstimulation (six or more contractions in 10 minutes), or hypertonus (single contraction lasting more than 2 minutes)."[1] Further adding to the confusion, the ACOG definitions are different from those used by many obstetric nurses, who commonly rely on the definitions provided by the Association of Women's Health, Obstetric and Neonatal Nurses (AWHONN).

AWHONN uses the term *hyperstimulus* and defines it as "contractions that occur more frequently than every 2 minutes; uterine relaxation less than 30 seconds between contractions; or uterine contractions that continue longer than 90-120 seconds."[5, p.149] AWHONN defines *hypertonus* in a variety of ways as well, including uterine resting tone of greater than 20 to 25 mm Hg, contractions peaking at greater than 80 mm Hg without pushing efforts, or more than 400 Montevideo units.[5, p.149] Because of the multitude of varying definitions in the literature and the fact that many of the definitions are incomplete (i.e., frequency alone with no clarification regarding intensity or duration and no differentiation between the first and second stages), it is no surprise that clinicians are confused. Fetal heart rate nomenclature is now standardized, so perhaps it is time for professional organizations to come together and standardize terms for uterine activity and uterine assessment as well. Until that becomes reality, institutions would be wise to reach consensus internally and adopt departmental policies that provide standard definitions for these terms. Inconsistent or incomplete definitions with regard to uterine activity can lead to miscommunication and error, and can create medico-legal problems should clinicians find themselves involved in litigation. For a more thorough discussion of the problems with use of inconsistent terms in fetal monitoring, see Chapter 10.

Clinicians need not wait for professional organizations to publish standardized definitions. The information in Box 4-2 can be used by clinicians and multidisciplinary committees to reach consensus on definitions for terms related to uterine activity. Based on a review of the physiology of normal uterine activity during labor (discussed in the preceding section) and uterine activity levels associated with fetal acidemia, as well as a review of the historical and current usage and definitions of terms related to uterine activity, this information should serve as the starting point for the development of clear, physiologically sound, and clinically useful definitions for terms related to excessive uterine activity. It is meant as an adjunct to, and not a replacement of, guidelines published by professional organizations.

A common claim in obstetric malpractice cases in both the U.S. and abroad is the inappropriate management of oxytocin-induced hyperstimulation.[16] Clinicians must work together, keeping patient safety the primary focus, and develop and encourage the use of standardized definitions for both normal and excessive uterine activity. In order to do so it is imperative to review the known physiologic aspects of uterine activity in normal labor, uterine activity associated with fetal acidemia, and both the current and historical definitions related to uterine activity. The desired result would be the development of sound practice guidelines that promote optimal uterine activity in labor without hyperstimulation.

Some clinicians contend that terms such as *hyperstimulation* should only apply when there are untoward fetal heart rate characteristics present, such as late decelerations. Not only is this in conflict with ACOG,[2] Bakker and colleagues[6] found no difference in the occurrence of late decelerations between the acidemic and non-acidemic fetuses, suggesting that the key to avoiding acidemia is not dependent upon the appearance of fetal heart rate changes, but rather the presence of excessive uterine activity itself. *Waiting to respond to excessive uterine activity until there are significant changes in fetal heart rate is not appropriate.* Rather, to prevent

BOX 4-2 Terms Related to Uterine Activity During Labor

Preliminary assumptions	■ Normal UA in first stage labor generally does not exceed 250 MVUs ■ Normal UA in second stage labor should not exceed 400 MVUs ■ Normal contraction duration generally ranges from 45 to 90 seconds ■ Normal contraction intensity (peak less resting tone) generally ranges from 25 to 80 mm Hg, with higher intensities common as labor progresses ■ Normal uterine resting tone ranges from 8 to 12 mm Hg and is generally not greater than 20 mm Hg
Tachysystole	■ Spontaneous occurrence of five or more uterine contractions of normal duration and intensity in 10 minutes in two or more consecutive 10-minute intervals ■ Spontaneous occurrence of uterine contractions that have a duration of greater than 90 seconds ■ Less than 30 to 60 seconds uterine relaxation between contractions (end of one contraction to onset of next)
Hyperstimulation	■ Presumes use of some type of cervical ripening agent or labor stimulant, such as oxytocin ■ Occurrence of five or more uterine contractions of normal duration and intensity in 10 minutes in two or more consecutive 10-minute intervals ■ Greater than 250 MVUs in first stage labor, greater than 400 MVUs in second stage labor ■ Occurrence of uterine contractions that have a duration of greater than 90 seconds ■ Less than 30 to 60 seconds uterine relaxation between contractions (end of one contraction to onset of next)
Hypertonus	■ Uterine resting tone of greater than 20 to 25 mm Hg or failure of the uterus to return to soft to palpation when acontractile.

Data from references 1, 2, 5, 6, 8-13, 15, 17, 18, 21, 22, 33, 34.

fetal acidemia at birth, clinicians should focus on *identifying and promoting normal (adequate) uterine activity* and correcting underlying causes of excessive uterine activity, whether it is *tachysystole, hyperstimulation, or hypertonus* (Figure 4-5).

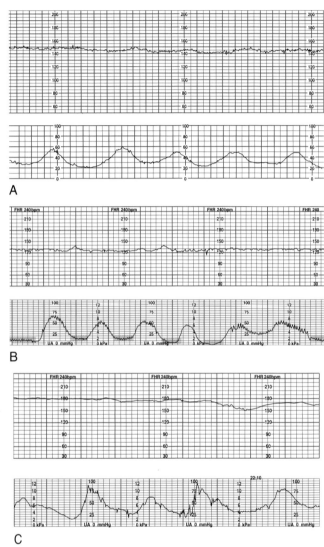

FIGURE 4-5 Examples of *tachysystole, hyperstimulation,* and *hypertonus.*
A. *Tachysystole* in a patient experiencing placental abruption. The patient was
later delivered by cesarean section and placental inspection confirmed an
approximately 40% abruption. **B.** *Hyperstimulation* in a patient whose labor is
being augmented with oxytocin. A tocotransducer is recording these
contractions, which were palpated as moderate to strong by the nurse. Note the
limited rest time between contractions (*highlighted areas*). **C.** *Hypertonus* and
hyperstimulation in a patient undergoing labor induction with oxytocin.
(Courtesy Lisa A. Miller, CNM, JD.)

Common Underlying Causes of Excessive Uterine Activity

- Use of pharmacologic cervical ripening agents
- Use of synthetic oxytocin for augmentation or induction (more common with high-dose, high-frequency administration protocols)
- Abruptio placentae
- Uterine over-distension, whether iatrogenic from amnioinfusion or as a result of multiple gestation, hydramnios, or macrosomia

Interventions to Decrease Excessive Uterine Activity

1. Change maternal position to lateral side-lying.
2. Administer a bolus of intravenous fluids and/or increase the maintenance IV rate.
3. Remove cervical ripening agents or, in the case of oxytocin usage, decrease or discontinue the infusion.
4. If excessive uterine activity related to the use of cervical ripening agents or oxytocin administration is noted in association with FHR changes indicative of hypoxemia, clinicians may consider the use of β2-adrenergic drugs (hexoprenaline or terbutaline).[1]

These interventions are specific to excessive uterine activity. Note that the management of fetal heart rate patterns is addressed in detail in Chapter 6. It is imperative that clinicians respond appropriately to fetal heart rate changes regardless of the nature of uterine activity, as uterine activity is only one of several causes of disrupted fetal oxygenation. But fetal heart rate changes are not a prerequisite for clinicians to respond to excessive uterine activity. Again, excessive uterine activity should trigger clinician response *whether or not fetal heart rate changes are observed.*

DIAGNOSIS AND MANAGEMENT OF LABOR ABNORMALITIES

Labor abnormalities may be described by clinicians using a variety of expressions, such as "slow progress in labor," "failure to progress," "dystocia," "dysfunctional labor," or "cephalopelvic disproportion."[20] Up to 68% of unanticipated cesarean deliveries in patients with vertex presentation are reported to be due to dystocia, and given the number of repeat cesarean deliveries that follow a primary cesarean for dystocia, the diagnosis of dystocia may account for as many as 60% of all cesarean births.[20] Strategies that have been shown to decrease the risk of dystocia include the following:[19,20,29]

- Avoidance of elective induction with an unripe cervix
- Avoidance of hospital admission during latent phase labor
- Upright maternal position
- Provision of continuous labor support
- Adequate maternal hydration
- Judicious use of epidural anesthesia

While a detailed discussion of the diagnosis and management of dystocia is outside the scope of this book, a brief overview is warranted and can be helpful when discussing management of uterine activity, especially when utilizing oxytocin, the most common treatment for dystocia.

Latent Phase Abnormalities

Labor is defined as "the presence of uterine contractions of sufficient intensity, frequency, and duration to bring about demonstrable effacement and dilation of the cervix."[2] While most clinicians agree that active phase labor begins when cervical dilation reaches 3 to 4 cm, there is little consensus regarding the definition for latent phase labor.[2,7,20,29] The most prevalent definition in clinical use is where the onset of labor to the beginning of active phase is considered the latent phase of labor.[20] Latent phase is considered prolonged if it is ≥20 hours in nulliparous patients and ≥14 hours in multiparous patients.[20] Considerations for the management of prolonged latent phase labor are listed next.

*Management Strategies for Latent Phase Disorders**

1. Avoid admission to the labor unit in latent phase labor. Unless otherwise indicated, admit only if the cervix is ≥3 cm dilated or 100% effaced. Educate patients antenatally about the benefits of this approach.
2. Assess the women's level of fatigue, and provide appropriate labor support.
3. Encourage adequate fluid intake and small, frequent meals while the mother is at home.
4. Set specific intervals to re-evaluate status, even if symptoms remain unchanged.

---

*Adapted from references 2, 19, 20, 30, 32.

5. Encourage ambulation to provide comfort and increase tolerance to latent phase labor.
6. Diagnose prolonged latent phase *only* after the presence of adequate UA for ≥ 20 hours in nulliparas and ≥ 14 hours in multiparas.
7. Provide adequate time for latent phase labor to progress during induction of labor. This may mean up to 18 hours in nulliparous women.
8. If induction is medically indicated, evaluate patients for appropriate methods of cervical ripening.
9. Unless medically indicated, avoid induction of labor, especially in the nulliparous patient with an unfavorable cervix.

Active Phase Abnormalities

Active phase labor abnormalities can be divided into three main categories:

1. *Protraction disorders:* a slow rate of cervical dilation, defined as less than the fifth percentile statistically
2. *Arrest disorders:* where labor progresses normally initially in active phase, then stops, for a period of at least 2 hours
3. *Combined disorders:* where slow progress precedes arrest[20]

ACOG recommends that oxytocin augmentation be considered for these disorders, stating that the goal "is to effect uterine activity sufficient to produce cervical change and fetal descent while avoiding uterine hyperstimulation and fetal compromise."[2] While traditionally the diagnosis of an arrest disorder required 2 hours without cervical change in the presence of a uterine contraction pattern that exceeded 200 Montevideo units,[2] studies[23,24,29] now suggest that 4 hours of uterine activity exceeding 200 Montevideo units (or 6 hours if the average uterine activity pattern was less than 200 Montevideo units) will result in up to a 92% vaginal delivery rate with no increased risk to the newborn. The suggested management approaches for active phase disorders are listed next.

*Management Strategies for Active Phase Disorders**

1. Ensure that cervix is dilated at least to 4 cm before diagnosing an active phase disorder.
2. Utilize low-dose, low-frequency oxytocin to achieve adequate UA while avoiding hyperstimulation.

---

*Adapted from references 2, 20, 23-29, 32, 33.

3. Consider an increase in the amount of hourly intravenous fluids to improve uterine muscle performance.
4. Consider use of an IUPC to document adequacy of contractions; a minimum of 200 Montevideo units is required.
5. Consider amniotomy if membranes are intact.
6. Limit active management of labor to nulliparas with singleton, cephalic presentations and normal FHR tracing components.
7. Require at least 4 hours of adequate UA before the diagnosis of failure to progress.
8. Provide continuous labor support.

Second Stage Abnormalities

Arrest of descent, failure of the fetus to rotate and descend, is the labor abnormality associated with the second stage. ACOG[2] considers the second stage prolonged in the nullipara if it exceeds 3 hours when regional anesthesia is being utilized, 2 hours if not. In the multipara, a second stage with regional anesthesia that is longer than 2 hours is considered prolonged; in the absence of regional anesthesia, it is 1 hour. Contrary to some clinicians' practices, these time frames are not mandates for delivery by cesarean section, but rather parameters for guiding assessment and intervention. Prolonged second stage should trigger clinical re-evaluation of the three P's: powers, passenger, and passage.[2] Evaluation of adequacy of uterine contractions, fetal position, and pelvic diameters may provide direction regarding interventions to facilitate rotation and descent.

UTERINE ACTIVITY AND OXYTOCIN USE

Oxytocin is a frequent treatment choice for labor abnormalities, and allegations related to oxytocin management are common in litigation.[16] There are many sound, evidence-based protocols for the administration of oxytocin, ranging from high-dose, high-frequency to low-dose, low-frequency, and hybrids that combine aspects of both regimens. Because oxytocin usage can result in excessive uterine activity, or *hyperstimulation*, it is important to closely and accurately monitor uterine activity when administering oxytocin.

Several studies[14,26-28] regarding the pharmacologic characteristics of oxytocin use in relation to dysfunctional labor and dystocia show that 40 minutes are needed to achieve maximum dose level.

Reviews by Arias[4] and Sanchez Ramos[25] regarding oxytocin pharmokinetics conclude that lower doses and less frequent increases of oxytocin are preferable, as they allow time for a more physiologic approach and avoid the risk of hyperstimulation associated with higher doses and shorter dosing intervals. Simpson and Creehan[31,33] suggest starting doses of 0.5 to 2 mU/min with increases every 30 to 60 minutes of 1 to 2 mU/min. This approach is in keeping with one of the primary tenets of pharmacology, which is *use the lowest amount of drug needed to achieve the desired effect.* Suggestions for the safe and effective use of oxytocin in labor are summarized in Box 4-3.

Oxytocin dosage should be titrated to uterine activity, with a goal of attaining adequate or normal uterine activity. *Coupling or tripling* of uterine contractions (Figure 4-6) is a phenomenon that may be seen with dysfunctional labor. Suggested treatment for this pattern is temporary discontinuation of oxytocin, lateral positioning of the mother, initiation of a fluid bolus, and a restart of oxytocin after 30 minutes or more.[33]

Uterine activity patterns reaching Montevideo units of 200 to 250 are an appropriate goal when administering oxytocin and utilizing internal monitoring. When external monitoring and palpation are being used, palpable contractions of normal duration every 2.5 to

---

BOX 4-3 Suggestions for Safe, Effective Oxytocin Use

- Utilize isotonic intravenous fluids during oxytocin administration to avoid dilutional hyponatremia.
- Administer oxytocin using a low-dose, low-frequency protocol to maximize pharmacologic dose response and avoid hyperstimulation.
- Use standardized definitions for the terms *adequate UA, hyperstimulation,* and *hypertonus,* and ensure that all team members are in accord.
- Resolve any episodes of hyperstimulation, regardless of whether or not FHR changes are present. Note that the goal of oxytocin use is *adequate* but not *excessive* UA.
- Once an adequate pattern of UA has been established, wean the oxytocin to the lowest amount necessary to maintain adequate contractions.
- If coupling and tripling of uterine contractions occur, discontinue oxytocin for 30 to 60 minutes, administer an intravenous fluid bolus (isotonic), and encourage the woman to adopt a side-lying position.

Data from references 2, 3, 16, 25-34.

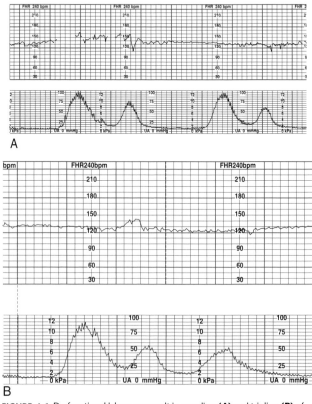

FIGURE 4-6 Dysfunctional labor may result in coupling **(A)** and tripling **(B)** of uterine contractions. Treatment consists of discontinuation of oxytocin, maternal position change, and intravenous hydration. (Courtesy Lisa A. Miller, CNM, JD.)

3 minutes should correlate well with adequate Montevideo units (Figure 4-7). If labor progress is not occurring with what appears to be adequate uterine activity to palpation, the proper clinical response *is to consider internal monitoring to more accurately assess uterine activity and **not** to increase the oxytocin.*

Hyperstimulation from oxytocin is a fairly common occurrence, even when using low-dose, low-frequency protocols. A sample management algorithm for hyperstimulation related to oxytocin use is presented in Figure 4-8. Continuous and ongoing evaluation of fetal status using a systematic approach can prevent fetal acidemia and reduce medical-legal risk. This can be achieved by avoidance of

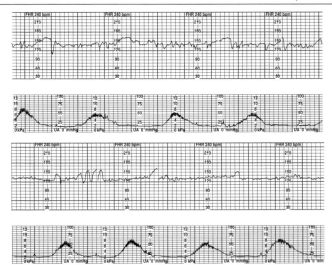

FIGURE 4-7 Example of adequate UA during oxytocin augmentation using external monitoring. Note adequate rest time between contractions. Contractions palpated as moderate according to nursing documentation. (Courtesy Lisa A. Miller, CNM, JD.)

injudicious use of oxytocin, adherence to guidelines regarding oxytocin titration, and appropriate team management of hyperstimulation.

SUMMARY

As Bakker[6] so aptly states, "contraction monitoring deserves full attention." Excessive uterine activity is related to fetal acidemia at birth and should be avoided by careful monitoring and judicious use of labor stimulants when necessary. Parameters for normal, or adequate, uterine activity are easily defined based on the physiology of normal labor. Clinicians must reach consensus on definitions related to excessive uterine activity and utilize standardized terminology for uterine activity in a fashion similar to that of standardized nomenclature for fetal heart rate patterns.

Understanding both the normal progress of labor and labor abnormalities is crucial to the promotion of improved outcomes for both mother and fetus. Continuous labor support, patient education regarding appropriate admission criteria, and adequate hydration play key roles in minimizing labor abnormalities. An understanding of the

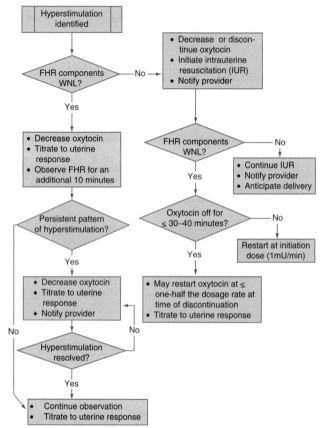

FIGURE 4-8 Sample management algorithm for treatment of hyperstimulation. (Adapted from hyperstimulation graphic. Mercy Medical Center, North Iowa, courtesy Amy Thorland.)

pharmacologic characteristics of oxytocin, combined with a focus on attaining adequate uterine activity, leads to safe and effective use of this common labor medication.

The evaluation of uterine activity and fetal heart rate patterns are inextricably intertwined in the care and support of the laboring mother. Focus on uterine activity assessment and management has been inconsistent in clinical practice. It is now clear that proper and careful assessment of uterine activity deserves consideration equal to that given to fetal heart rate pattern assessment.

References

1. American College of Obstetricians and Gynecologists: Intrapartum fetal heart rate monitoring. ACOG *Practice Bulletin* no.70, *Obstet Gynecol* 106(6):1453-1460, 2005.

2. American College of Obstetricians and Gynecologists: *Dystocia and augmentation of labor,* Practice Bulletin no. 49, Washington, DC, December, 2003 (*reaffirmed September 2006*), ACOG.

3. American College of Obstetricians and Gynecologists: *Induction of labor,* Practice Bulletin no. 10, November 1999, ACOG.

4. Arias F: Pharmacology of oxytocin and prostaglandins. *Clin Obstet Gynecol* 43(3):455-468, 2000.

5. Association of Women's Health, Obstetric and Neonatal Nurses (AWHONN): *Fetal heart monitoring: Principles and practices*, ed 3, Dubuque, Iowa, 2003, Kendall/Hunt.

6. Bakker PCAM, Kurver PHJ, Kuik DJ, Van Geijn HP: Elevated uterine activity increases the risk of fetal acidosis at birth. *Am J Obstet Gynecol* 196(4):313,e1-e6, 2007.

7. Beckmann M: Predicting a failed induction. *Aust N Z J Obstet Gynaecol* 47(5):394-398, 2007.

8. Caldeyro-Barcia R: Intrauterine fetal reanimation in acute intrapartum fetal distress. *Early Hum Dev* 29:27-33, 1992.

9. Caldeyro-Barcia R: Oxytocin in pregnancy and labour. *Acta Endocrinol Suppl (Copenh)* 34(Suppl 50):41-49, 1960.

10. Caldeyro-Barcia R, Poseiro JJ: Oxytocin and contractility of the pregnant human uterus. *Ann N Y Acad Sci* 75:813-830, 1959.

11. Caldeyro-Barcia R, Poseiro JJ: Physiology of uterine contractions. *Clin Obstet Gynecol* 3:386-408, 1960.

12. Caldeyro-Barcia R, Sica-Blanco Y, Poseiro JJ, Gonzalez Panizza V, Mendez-Bauer C, Fielitz C, Alvarez H, Pose S, Hendricks C: A quantitative study of the action of synthetic oxytocin on the pregnant human uterus. *J Pharmacol Exp Ther* 121(1):18-31, 1957.

13. Caldeyro-Barcia R, Theobald G: Sensitivity of the pregnant human myometrium to oxytocin. *Am J Obstet Gynecol* 102(8):1181, 1968.

14. Crall HD, Mattison DR: Oxytocin pharmacodynamics: Effect of long infusions on uterine activity. *Gynecol Obstet Invest* 31(1):17-22, 1991.

15. Effer SB, Bértola RP, Vrettos A, Caldeyro-Barcia R: Quantitative study of the regularity of uterine contractile rhythm in labor. *Am J Obstet Gynecol* 105(6):909-915, 1969.

16. Jonsson M, Nordén SL, Hanson U: Analysis of malpractice claims with a focus on oxytocin use in labour. *Acta Obstetricia et Gynecologica Scandanavica* 86(3):315-319, 2007.

17. Krapohl AJ, Myers GG, Caldeyro-Barcia R: Uterine contractions in spontaneous labor. A quantitative study. *Am J Obstet Gynecol* 106(3): 378-387, 1970.

18. Lowdermilk DL, Perry SE: *Maternity & women's health care*, ed 9, St Louis, 2007, Mosby.

19. Mercer BM: Induction of labor in the nulliparous gravida with an unfavorable cervix. *Obstet Gynecol* 105(4):688-689, 2005.

20. Ness A, Goldberg J, Berghella V: Abnormalities of the first and second stages of labor. *Obstet Gynecol Clin N Am*, 32(2):201-220, 2005.

21. Peebles D, Spencer J, Edwards A, Wyatt J, Reynolds E, Cope M, Delpy D: Relation between frequency of uterine contractions and human fetal cerebral oxygenation saturation studied during labour by near infrared spectroscopy. *Br J Obstet Gynaecol* 101(1):44-48, 1994.

22. Pontonnier G, Puech F, Grandjean H, Rolland M: Some physical and biochemical parameters during normal labour. *Biol Neonate* 26(3-4): 159-173, 1975.

23. Rouse DJ, Owen J, Hauth JC: Criteria for failed labor induction: prospective evaluation of a standardized protocol. *Obstet Gynecol* 96(5 Pt 1):671-677, 2000.

24. Rouse D, Owen J, Savage K, Hauth J: Active phase labor arrest: Revisiting the 2-hour minimum. *Obstet Gynecol* 98(4):550-554, 2001.

25. Sanchez-Ramos L: Induction of labor. *Obstet Gynecol Clin North Am* 32(2):181-200, 2005.

26. Seitchik J: The management of functional dystocia in the first stage of labor. *Clin Obstet Gynecol* 30(1):42-49, 1987.

27. Seitchik J, Amico JA, Castillo M, Oxytocin augmentation of dysfunctional labor. V. An alternative oxytocin regimen. *Am J Obstet Gynecol* 151(6):757-761, 1985.

28. Seitchik J, Amico J, Robinson AG, Castillo M: Oxytocin augmentation of dysfunctional labor. IV. Oxytocin pharmacokinetics. *Am J Obstet Gynecol* 150(3):225-228, 1984.

29. Shields S, Ratcliffe S, Fontaine P, Leeman L: Dystocia in nulliparous women. *Am Fam Physician* 75(11):1671-1678, 2007.

30. Simon C, Grobman W: When has an induction failed? *Obstet Gynecol* 105(4):705-709, 2005.

31. Simpson KR: *Cervical ripening and induction and augmentation of labor*, ed 2, Washington, DC, 2002, Association of Women's Health, Obstetric and Neonatal Nurses.

32. Simpson KR: Intrauterine resuscitation during labor: Review of current methods and supportive evidence. *J Midwifery Womens Health* 52(3):229-237, 2007.

33. Simpson KR, Creehan PA: *Perinatal nursing*, ed 3, Philadelphia, 2008, Lippincott Williams & Wilkins.

34. Simpson KR, James DC, Knox GE: Nurse-physician communication during labor and birth: implications for patient safety. *J Obstet Gynecol Neonatal Nurs* 35(4):547-556, 2006.

CHAPTER 5

Pattern Recognition and Interpretation

The clinical application of electronic fetal heart rate (FHR) monitoring consists of three separate but interdependent elements: terminology, interpretation, and management.

Terminology(n.) The vocabulary of technical terms used in a particular field, subject, science, or art

Interpretation(n.) Establishing the meaning or significance of something

Management(n.) The act of handling or controlling something successfully

This chapter addresses the standardized terminology used to define fetal heart rate patterns and the interpretation of fetal heart rate patterns with respect to underlying physiology. The principles developed in this chapter are used in the discussion of fetal heart rate management that follows in Chapter 6.

THE EVOLUTION OF STANDARDIZED FETAL HEART RATE TERMINOLOGY

Electronic fetal heart rate monitoring was introduced into clinical practice before consensus was achieved regarding standardized terminology. This resulted in wide variations in the description and interpretation of common fetal heart rate patterns. Lack of standardization was a major impediment to effective communication. In 1995 and 1996, the National Institute of Child Health and Human Development (NICHD) convened a workshop to develop "standardized and unambiguous definitions for fetal heart rate tracings".[31] Recommendations from the workshop were published in 1997 in both the *American Journal of Obstetrics and Gynecology* and in the *Journal of Obstetric, Gynecologic, and Neonatal Nurses*. However, the NICHD recommendations were not incorporated rapidly into clinical practice and wide variations persisted. In May 2005, the American College of Obstetricians and Gynecologists (ACOG) endorsed the 1997 NICHD recommendations in *Practice Bulletin* no. 62, titled "Intrapartum Fetal Heart Rate Monitoring" (subsequently updated in December 2005, *Practice Bulletin* no. 70).[2] Shortly after ACOG issued *Practice Bulletin* no. 62, the Association of Women's Health, Obstetric and Neonatal Nurses (AWHONN) endorsed the NICHD terminology stating "AWHONN's decision is based on recognition of the importance of ensuring the use of standardized terminology among health care providers to communicate fetal heart monitoring and promote patient safety".[4] In December 2006, the American College of Nurse-Midwives (ACNM) issued a position statement[1] encouraging the use of NICHD nomenclature as the standard when using electronic fetal monitoring. For the first time since electronic fetal heart rate monitoring was introduced, professional organizations representing providers of obstetric care in the United States (ACOG, AWHONN, ACNM) had reached consensus regarding a standardized set of definitions for fetal heart rate patterns. The standardized NICHD fetal heart rate definitions published in 1997 are summarized in Box 5-1. Detailed discussion of individual pattern definitions, along with evidence-based review of the underlying fetal physiology, is presented later in this chapter.

EVIDENCE-BASED INTERPRETATION OF FETAL HEART RATE PATTERNS

The fetal physiology underlying common fetal heart rate patterns has been the subject of scientific investigation for at least four decades. Many of the principles that are taught and promulgated are based on sound scientific evidence. However, a surprising number of fetal heart rate "facts" have been handed down from generation to generation without the support of scientific evidence. Many of the fetal heart rate theories that pass for "facts" are based on plausible physiologic mechanisms; however, most have not been substantiated by systematic research. Others do not even reach the level of physiologic plausibility. In an area as critical as intrapartum fetal heart rate monitoring, it is imperative that care providers recognize the difference between practices that are based on sound scientific evidence and practices that are based on unsubstantiated theories. This chapter reviews the relationship between fetal physiology and fetal heart rate patterns with emphasis on the underlying

BOX 5-1 Standardized Fetal Heart Rate Definitions

Pattern	Definition
Baseline	Mean FHR rounded to increments of 5 bpm during a 10-min segment, excluding periodic or episodic changes, periods of marked variability, or segments of baseline that differ by >25 bpm
	The baseline must be at least 2 min in any 10-min segment (not necessarily contiguous)
	Normal baseline FHR range 110-160 bpm
	Baseline >160 bpm = tachycardia; baseline <110 bpm = bradycardia
Variability	Fluctuations in the FHR baseline of two cycles per min or greater
	Quantitated as the amplitude of peak-to-trough in bpm
	Absent – amplitude range undetectable
	Minimal – amplitude range detectable ≤ 5 bpm
	Moderate (normal) – amplitude range 6-25 bpm
	Marked – amplitude range >25 bpm
Accelerations	Abrupt increase (onset to peak <30 sec) in the FHR from the most recently calculated baseline
	At ≥32 weeks, an acceleration peaks ≥15 bpm above baseline and lasts ≥15 sec but <2 min
	At <32 weeks, an acceleration peaks ≥10 bpm above baseline and lasts ≥15 sec but <2 min
	Prolonged acceleration lasts ≥2 min, but< 10 min; acceleration ≥10 min is a baseline change
Decelerations	
Early	Gradual (onset to nadir ≥30 sec) decrease in FHR during a uterine contraction
	Nadir of the deceleration occurs at the same time as the peak of the contraction
Late	Gradual (onset to nadir ≥30 sec) decrease in FHR during a uterine contraction
	Onset, nadir, and recovery occur after the beginning, peak, and end of the contraction
Variable	Abrupt (onset to nadir < 0 sec) decrease in the FHR ≥15 bpm below the baseline lasting ≥15 sec but <2 min
Prolonged	Deceleration ≥15 bpm below baseline lasting ≥2 min or more but <10 min

scientific evidence. Principles of fetal heart rate interpretation are stratified by supporting evidence according to the method outlined by the U.S. Preventive Services Task Force (Box 5-2).[45] Level I evidence is considered to be the most robust and Level III, the least.

The *primary objective of intrapartum fetal heart rate monitoring is to provide information regarding fetal oxygenation during labor*, as discussed in Chapter 2. However, a number of different conditions and/or exposures can influence the appearance of a fetal heart rate tracing via mechanisms unrelated to fetal oxygenation. Common examples include maternal fever, fetal cardiac arrhythmias, medications, and fetal anemia. Thorough assessment of a fetal heart rate tracing must take in account all of the "differentials" summarized in Table 5-1. If a fetal heart rate abnormality is thought to be related to disrupted fetal oxygenation, management is directed at improving the transfer of oxygen from the environment to the fetus along the oxygen pathway, as described in Chapter 2. However, if a fetal heart rate abnormality is thought to be related to any of the maternal and fetal factors summarized in Table 5-1, *individualized management* is directed at the specific underlying cause. This concept is illustrated in Figure 5-1. During the following discussion of physiology and interpretation, *fetal heart rate patterns related to disrupted fetal oxygenation are considered separately from fetal heart rate patterns caused by other mechanisms.*

BOX 5-2   Stratification of Scientific Evidence*

Level I	Evidence obtained from at least one properly designed randomized controlled trial.
Level II-1	Evidence obtained from well-designed controlled trials without randomization.
Level II-2	Evidence obtained from well-designed cohort or case–control analytic studies, preferably from more than one center or research group.
Level II-3	Evidence obtained from multiple time series with or without the intervention. Dramatic results in uncontrolled experiments also could be regarded as this type of evidence.
Level III	Opinions of respected authorities, based on clinical experience, descriptive studies, or reports of expert committees.

*According to method outlined by U.S. Preventive Services Task Force[45].

TABLE 5-1 "Differential" Factors not Specifically Related to Fetal Oxygenation that may Influence Fetal Heart Rate

Factor	Reported FHR Associations (Most Evidence is Level II-3 and Level III)
Prematurity	Increased baseline rate, decreased variability, reduced frequency and amplitude of accelerations
Sleep cycle	Decreased variability, reduced frequency and amplitude of accelerations
Fever/infection	Increased baseline rate, decreased variability
Medications	Effects depend upon specific medication and may include changes in baseline rate, frequency and amplitude of accelerations, variability, and sinusoidal pattern
Hyperthyroidism	Tachycardia, decreased variability
Fetal anemia	Sinusoidal pattern, tachycardia
Fetal heart block	Bradycardia, decreased variability
Fetal cardiac failure	Tachycardia, bradycardia, decreased variability
Maternal hypoglycemia	Bradycardia
Maternal hypothermia	Bradycardia
Fetal tachyarrhythmia	Variable degrees of tachycardia, decreased variability
Congenital anomaly	Decreased variability, decelerations
Preexisting neurologic abnormality	Decreased variability, absent accelerations

NATIONAL INSTITUTE OF CHILD HEALTH AND HUMAN DEVELOPMENT TERMINOLOGY: GENERAL CONSIDERATIONS

The standardized definitions proposed by the NICHD apply to the interpretation of fetal heart rate patterns produced by a direct fetal electrode detecting the fetal electrocardiogram or by an external Doppler device detecting fetal cardiac motion using the autocorrelation technique. Autocorrelation is a computerized method of minimizing the artifact associated with Doppler ultrasound calculation of the fetal heart rate. This technology is built in to all modern fetal heart rate monitors.

Other general considerations are as follows:

- Patterns are categorized as baseline, periodic, or episodic.
- Baseline patterns include baseline rate and variability.
- Periodic and episodic patterns include FHR accelerations and decelerations.

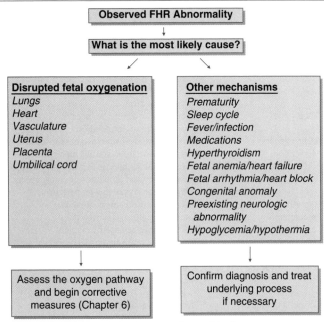

FIGURE 5-1 Stratifying FHR abnormalities by cause.

- Periodic patterns are those associated *with* uterine contractions.
- Episodic patterns are those *not* associated with uterine contractions.
- Deceleration onset is defined as *abrupt* if the onset to nadir (lowest point) is less than 30 seconds and *gradual* if the onset to nadir is 30 seconds or greater.
- Although terms such as *beat-to-beat* variability, *short-term* variability, and *long-term* variability are used frequently in clinical practice, the NICHD panel recommended that no distinction be made between *short-term* or *beat-to-beat* variability, and *long-term* variability because in actual practice they are visually determined as a unit.
- A number of FHR characteristics are dependent upon gestational age, so gestational age must be considered in the full evaluation of the pattern. In addition, the FHR tracing should be evaluated in the context of maternal medical condition, prior results of fetal assessment, medications, and other factors.

- It is essential to recognize that FHR patterns do not occur alone and generally evolve over time. Therefore, a full description of a FHR tracing requires a qualitative and quantitative description of each of the five essential FHR components listed below.

FIVE BASIC COMPONENTS OF A FETAL HEART RATE TRACING

The *five basic components* of a fetal heart rate tracing are:
1. Baseline rate
2. Baseline variability
3. Accelerations
4. Decelerations
5. Changes or trends over time

TERMINOLOGY, PHYSIOLOGY, AND INTERPRETATION OF SPECIFIC FETAL HEART RATE PATTERNS

BASELINE RATE

Definition

Baseline fetal heart rate is defined as the approximate mean fetal heart rate rounded to increments of 5 beats per minute (bpm) during a 10-minute segment, excluding periodic or episodic changes, periods of marked variability, and segments of baseline that differ by more than 25 beats per minute (Figure 5-2). Normal fetal heart rate baseline ranges from 110 to 160 beats per minute. In any 10-minute window, the minimum baseline duration must be at least 2 minutes or the baseline for that period is deemed indeterminate. The definition does not mandate that the 2 minutes be contiguous.

The baseline rate is reported as a single number (e.g., 145 beats per minute), not as a range (e.g., 140-150 beats per minute or 140s). This is a fundamental principle of fetal heart rate terminology, because the definitions of other fetal heart rate components, including accelerations and decelerations, are based on the degree of deviation from the baseline rate. If the baseline during any 10-minute segment is deemed indeterminate, it may be necessary to refer to

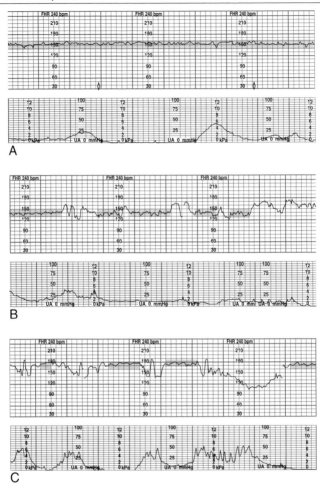

FIGURE 5-2 FHR baseline. Note that the 2-minute minimum for identifiable baseline does not require 2 contiguous or continuous minutes; rather it is the total identifiable baseline in the 10-minute window that must add up to 2 minutes. Also, baseline may occur (and be interpreted) during contractions, as seen in example A. **A.** Baseline *(highlighted)* is identified over entire 10-minute window, exceeding the 2-minute minimum. **B.** Baseline *(highlighted)* is identified between accelerations or between segments differing by 25 bpm or more; identifiable baseline is approximately 5 minutes total (note the 2-minute minimum is met). **C.** Baseline *(highlighted)* is identified between decelerations or between segments differing by 25 bpm or more; identifiable baseline is approximately 5 minutes total (note the 2-minute minimum is met).

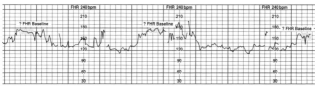

FHR baseline here is indeterminate. There is not enough identifiable baseline to meet the 2-minute minimum. Prior baseline was 155 bpm.

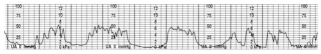

FIGURE 5-3 Indeterminate baseline. Note that there are less than 2 minutes of identifiable baseline during this 10-minute window. The baseline would be labeled "indeterminate" for this portion of the tracing, and the clinician would need to refer to previous portions of the strip to determine baseline. FHR baseline is indeterminate. There is not enough identifiable baseline to meet the 2-minute minimum. Prior baseline was 155 bpm.

previous 10-minute segment(s) for determination of the baseline (Figure 5-3).

Physiology

Baseline fetal heart rate is regulated by intrinsic cardiac pacemakers (sinoatrial node, atrioventricular [AV] node) and conduction pathways, autonomic innervation (sympathetic, parasympathetic), humoral factors (catecholamines), extrinsic factors (medications) and local factors (calcium, potassium). Sympathetic innervation and plasma catecholamines increase baseline fetal heart rate while parasympathetic innervation reduces the baseline rate. Autonomic input regulates the fetal heart rate in response to fluctuations in P_{O_2} (partial pressure of oxygen), P_{CO_2} (partial pressure of carbon dioxide), and blood pressure detected by chemoreceptors and baroreceptors located in the aortic arch and carotid arteries.

CATEGORIES OF BASELINE RATE

TACHYCARDIA

Definition

Baseline fetal heart rate in excess of 160 beats per minute is defined as tachycardia (Figure 5-4). Tachycardia is quantitated as the

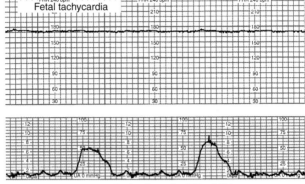

FIGURE 5-4 Fetal tachycardia: FHR >160 bpm.

approximate mean fetal heart rate in beats per minute, rounded to the nearest 5 BPM.

Interpretation

Fetal oxygenation: As discussed in Chapter 2, recurrent or sustained disruption of oxygen transfer from the environment to the fetus can lead to progressive deterioration of fetal oxygenation and, eventually, to fetal metabolic acidemia. In the setting of metabolic acidemia, blunting of parasympathetic cardiac stimulation can cause the fetal heart rate to rise above the normal range. Sympathetic and humoral factors may play a role as well. In the setting of recurrent fetal heart rate decelerations, a rising fetal heart rate baseline may indicate that disruption of fetal oxygenation has progressed to the stage of metabolic acidemia, particularly if other components of the fetal heart rate tracing are abnormal (absent variability, absent accelerations).

There are many other potential causes of fetal tachycardia; therefore, the relationship between fetal tachycardia and fetal oxygenation is nonspecific. While the physiologic basis is sound, the scientific evidence supporting a relationship between fetal tachycardia and disrupted oxygenation is primarily Level III. Nevertheless, the observation of fetal tachycardia should prompt consideration of all possible causes, including disrupted oxygenation that has progressed to the stage of metabolic acidemia.

Other mechanisms: Fetal tachycardia can be caused by many mechanisms that are unrelated to fetal oxygenation. For example, abnormalities involving fetal cardiac pacemakers and/or the cardiac conduction system can result in sinus tachycardia, supraventricular tachycardia, atrial fibrillation, atrial flutter, and ventricular dysrhythmias. Maternal fever, infection, and fetal anemia are well-known associations that likely act through the fetal autonomic nervous system and circulating factors (catecholamines) to cause fetal tachycardia. Increased fetal oxygen consumption and/or decreased fetal oxygen carrying capacity might contribute to the physiologic changes observed in these settings. However, reduced fetal oxygenation is not the initiating factor.

In the setting of extreme prematurity (prior to viability), a baseline fetal heart rate in excess of 160 beats per minute may have no specific clinical significance. Maternal thyroid stimulating antibodies can cause maternal hyperthyroidism and maternal tachycardia. Rarely, transplacental passage of thyroid stimulating antibodies can result in fetal hyperthyroidism and tachycardia. Finally, many medications have been reported to cause fetal tachycardia. General categories include parasympatholytic drugs (atropine, hydroxyzine, phenothiazines) and sympathomimetic drugs (terbutaline, ritodrine, albuterol). Caffeine, theophylline, cocaine, and methamphetamine are other possible causes. All of the associations mentioned above are physiologically plausible, but few have been subjected to prospective analysis. Virtually all of the scientific evidence regarding these mechanisms is Level II-3 and Level III.

Causes of fetal tachycardia (evidence Level II-3 and Level III) include the following:

Causes Related to Fetal Oxygenation

- Progressive disruption of fetal oxygenation leading to metabolic acidemia
- Blunted autonomic regulation of the FHR

Other Mechanisms

- Tachyarrhythmias
    Sinus tachycardia
    Supraventricular tachycardia
    Atrial fibrillation
    Atrial flutter
    Ventricular dysrhythmias
- Maternal fever
- Infection (including chorioamnionitis)
- Fetal anemia

- Hyperthyroidism
- Medications
    Sympathomimetics (terbutaline, ritodrine, albuterol)
    Parasympathetics (atropine, hydroxyzine, phenothiazines)
- Drugs
    Caffeine, theophylline
    Cocaine
    Methamphetamine

BRADYCARDIA

Definition

Baseline fetal heart rate less than 110 beats per minute is defined as bradycardia (Figure 5-5). Bradycardia is quantitated as the approximate mean fetal heart rate in beats per minute, rounded to the nearest 5 bpm.

Interpretation

Fetal oxygenation: In the past, some clinicians used the term *brady-cardia* interchangeably with *prolonged deceleration*. This practice is imprecise and should be avoided. According to the definitions published by the NICHD, bradycardia is a baseline rate below 110 beats per minute, whereas a prolonged deceleration is a periodic or episodic deceleration that interrupts the baseline. *The distinction is*

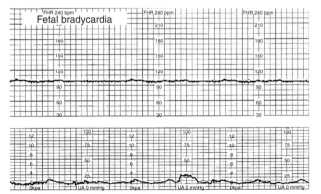

FIGURE 5-5 Fetal bradycardia: FHR <110 bpm.

critical. Decelerations are common and can reflect disrupted fetal oxygenation. On the other hand, true baseline bradycardia is rare and is not specifically related to fetal oxygenation.

Other mechanisms: True fetal bradycardia can be caused by abnormalities at the level of the cardiac pacemakers and/or conduction system. Atrioventricular dissociation or "heart block" can result from disruption of the cardiac conduction system by structural cardiac defects, viral infections (cytomegalovirus) or maternal Sjögren's antibodies. Medications (adrenergic antagonists) rarely cause a reduction in baseline fetal heart rate below 110 beats per minute. Fetal bradycardia has been described in association with fetal heart failure, maternal hypoglycemia and maternal hypothermia during cardiac surgery, urosepsis, and magnesium sulfate infusion. Most of the scientific evidence regarding these mechanisms is Level II-3 or Level III.

Causes of fetal bradycardia include the following:

Causes Related to Fetal Oxygenation

- Baseline FHR bradycardia alone is not specifically related to fetal oxygenation.
- The clinical significance of fetal bradycardia depends on the *underlying cause* and *accompanying* FHR patterns, including variability, accelerations, or decelerations.

Other Mechanisms

- AV dissociation (heart block)
- Structural defects
- Viral infections (e.g., cytomegalovirus)
- Sjögren's antibodies
- Medications
- Fetal heart failure
- Maternal hypoglycemia
- Maternal hypothermia

BASELINE FETAL HEART RATE VARIABILITY

Definition

Baseline fetal heart rate variability is defined as fluctuations in the baseline fetal heart rate of two cycles per minute or greater. The fluctuations are irregular in amplitude and frequency. Variability is quantitated in beats per minute and is measured from the peak to the trough of a single cycle. Variability is categorized as absent, minimal, moderate, or marked based on the amplitude range as summarized below.

Categories of Fetal Heart Rate Variability

- Absent: Amplitude range undetectable
- Minimal: Amplitude range detectable but ≤5 bpm
- Moderate: Amplitude range 6-25 bpm
- Marked: Amplitude range >25 bpm

No distinction is made between *short-term* (*beat-to-beat*) variability and *long-term* variability because in actual practice they are visually determined as a unit. There is no consensus whether "beat-to-beat" variability alone is interpretable to the unaided eye. The sinusoidal pattern has a smooth, sine wave-like pattern of regular frequency and amplitude. It is not included in the definition of fetal heart rate variability.

Physiology

Many factors interact to regulate fetal heart rate variability, including cardiac pacemakers (sinoatrial node, atrioventricular node) and the cardiac conduction system, autonomic innervation (sympathetic, parasympathetic), humoral factors (catecholamines), extrinsic factors (medications), and local factors (calcium, potassium). Fluctuations in Po_2, Pco_2, and blood pressure are detected by chemoreceptors and baroreceptors located in the aortic arch and carotid arteries. Signals from these receptors are processed in the medullary vasomotor center with regulatory input from higher centers in the hypothalamus and cerebral cortex. Sympathetic and parasympathetic signals from the medullary vasomotor center modulate the fetal heart rate in response to moment-to-moment changes in fetal Po_2, Pco_2, and blood pressure. With every heartbeat, slight corrections in the heart rate help to optimize fetal cardiac output and maximize the distribution of oxygenated blood to the fetal tissues. As explained in Chapter 3, this variation is referred to as fetal heart rate variability and is displayed visually on the fetal heart rate graph as an irregular horizontal line. The small oscillations that represent fetal heart rate changes between each successive heartbeat have been referred to as *beat-to-beat* variability or *short-term* variability. The broader oscillations that occur at least twice per minute have been referred to as *long-term* variability. These terms describe two essential physiologic elements of fetal heart rate variability that occur together and that are evaluated as a unit. Therefore, as discussed above, *no distinction is made between short-term (beat-to-beat) variability and long-term variability.* These terms are not included in standardized NICHD terminology and should be avoided.

CATEGORIES OF BASELINE VARIABILITY

Absent Variability

Definition

Variability is defined as absent when the amplitude range of the fetal heart rate fluctuations is undetectable to the unaided eye, as depicted in Figure 5-6.

Interpretation

Fetal oxygenation: Recurrent or sustained disruption of oxygen transfer from the environment to the fetus can lead to progressive deterioration of fetal oxygenation, metabolic acidemia, and blunting of parasympathetic outflow that can result in loss of moment-to-moment regulation of the fetal heart rate. In the fetal heart rate tracing, these changes can be seen as decreased variability. While fetal heart rate variability ≤5 beats per minute is relatively common,

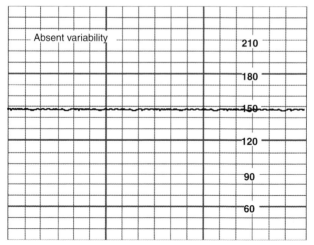

FIGURE 5-6 Absent variability: amplitude range undetectable.

persistently absent variability (amplitude range undetectable) is rare. If decreased variability is caused by disrupted fetal oxygenation, other components of the fetal heart rate tracing are frequently abnormal, including recurrent decelerations, absent accelerations, and tachycardia. There are many possible causes of decreased fetal heart rate variability (≤5 beats per minute). When persistent absent variability (amplitude range undetectable) is observed, careful evaluation should be undertaken to exclude fetal metabolic acidemia.

Other mechanisms: Other causes of persistent absent variability include congenital anomalies and preexisting neurologic injury. However, it is imperative that clinicians view the development of persistent absent variability during the intrapartum course as indicative of evolving fetal metabolic acidemia until proven otherwise.

Minimal Variability

Definition

Variability is defined as minimal when the amplitude range is detectable, but less than or equal to 5 beats per minute, as illustrated in Figure 5-7.

Interpretation

Fetal oxygenation: Disrupted fetal oxygenation leading to metabolic acidemia and blunting of the normal autonomic regulation

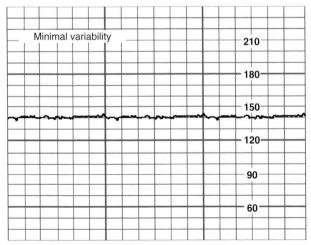

FIGURE 5-7 Minimal variability: amplitude range detectable ≤5 bpm.

of the fetal heart rate can result in decreased fetal heart rate variability. The specific relationship between minimal variability, fetal oxygenation, and fetal metabolic acidemia is not known, primarily because the literature has not consistently distinguished between minimal and absent variability. When minimal variability is observed, all possible causes should be considered, including disrupted fetal oxygenation and evolving metabolic acidemia.

Other mechanisms: Decreased fetal heart rate variability can be caused by a number of mechanisms that are unrelated to fetal oxygenation, including fetal sleep cycles, fetal tachycardia, and extreme prematurity. Congenital anomalies and preexisting neurologic injury are other possible causes. Several medications have been implicated in decreased fetal heart rate variability. General categories include central nervous system (CNS) depressants (narcotics, barbiturates, phenothiazines, tranquilizers, general anesthetics) and parasympatholytics (atropine). While all of these associations are biologically plausible, few have been subjected to prospective analysis. Most of the scientific evidence regarding these mechanisms is Level II-3 and Level III. It is important to note that most studies in the literature define decreased variability as ≤5 beats per minute and do not further stratify variability as absent (amplitude range undetectable) or minimal (amplitude range detectable but ≤5 beats per minute). Therefore, it is not possible to draw valid conclusions regarding the relative clinical significance of these two categories. Causes of decreased fetal heart rate variability are summarized below.

Causes of decreased variability (evidence Level II-3 and Level III) are as follows:

Causes Related to Fetal Oxygenation

- Progressive disruption of fetal oxygenation leading to metabolic acidemia
- Blunted autonomic regulation of the FHR

Other Mechanisms

- Fetal sleep cycles
- Fetal tachycardia
- Prematurity
- Congenital anomalies
- Preexisting neurologic injury
- Medications
- CNS depressants
    Narcotics

- CNS depressants (Cont.)
  - Barbiturates
  - Phenothiazines
  - Tranquilizers
  - General Anesthetics
- Parasympatholytics
  - Atropine
  - Phenothiazines

Moderate Variability

Definition

Variability is defined as moderate when the amplitude range of the fetal heart rate fluctuations is 6 to 25 beats per minute, as illustrated in Figure 5-8.

Interpretation

Fetal oxygenation: Moderate (normal) fetal heart rate variability indicates normal control of the fetal heart rate by cardiac pacemakers and conduction pathways, autonomic innervation, humoral, extrinsic, and local factors. Specifically, moderate variability indicates that autonomic regulation of the fetal heart rate is not blunted by disrupted fetal oxygenation that has progressed to the stage of metabolic acidemia. *One of the central concepts of electronic fetal heart*

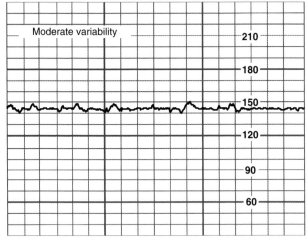

FIGURE 5-8 Moderate variability: amplitude range 6-25 bpm.

*rate monitoring is that moderate variability is highly predictive of the absence of fetal metabolic acidemia at the time it is observed.** Supporting evidence is Levels II-2, II-3, and III.

Other mechanisms: Moderate variability also indicates that fetal heart rate regulation is not significantly impacted by fetal sleep cycles, tachycardia, prematurity, congenital anomalies, preexisting neurologic injury, central nervous system depressants or parasym-patholytic medications.[14,16,17,47]

Marked Variability

Definition

Variability is defined as marked when the amplitude range of the fetal heart rate fluctuations is greater than 25 beats per minute as illustrated in Figure 5-9.

Interpretation

The significance of marked variability is not known. In many cases, it likely represents a normal variant. It is plausible that marked variability reflects autonomic perturbation in the setting of early hypoxemia. Scientific evidence regarding this pattern is limited. All available evidence is Level III.

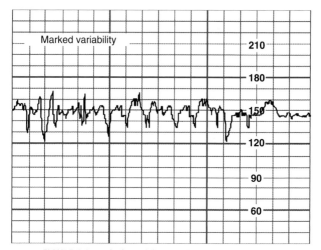

FIGURE 5-9 Marked variability: amplitude range >25 bpm.

*References 2,13,18,28,32,33

SINUSOIDAL PATTERN

Sinusoidal fetal heart rate is an uncommon pattern that is not included in the definition of fetal heart rate variability (Figure 5-10). The pattern is a smooth sine wave with regular frequency and amplitude. It is not a type of fetal heart rate variability.

Although the pathophysiologic mechanism is not known, this pattern classically is associated with severe fetal anemia. Variations of the pattern have been described in association with chorioamnionitis, fetal sepsis, or administration of narcotic analgesics.[17] Scientific evidence regarding the etiology of the sinusoidal pattern is Level II-2 to Level III. Evidence regarding pathophysiology is Level III.

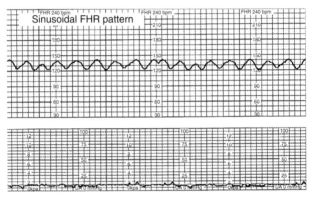

FIGURE 5-10 Sinusoidal pattern.

ACCELERATIONS

Definition

Acceleration is an abrupt (onset to peak <30 seconds) increase in fetal heart rate above the baseline, calculated from the most recently determined portion of the baseline. The peak is at least 15 beats per minute above the baseline and the acceleration lasts at least 15 seconds from the onset to return to baseline (Figure 5-11).

Before 32 weeks of gestation, an acceleration is defined as having a peak at least 10 beats per minute above the baseline and a duration of at least 10 seconds. An acceleration lasting at least 2 minutes but less than 10 minutes is defined as a prolonged acceleration. An acceleration lasting 10 minutes or longer is defined as a baseline

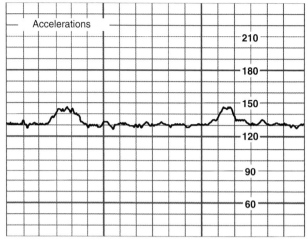

FIGURE 5-11 Accelerations.

change. The amplitude of an acceleration is quantitated in beats per minute above the baseline excluding transient spikes or electronic artifact. The duration is quantitated in minutes and seconds.

Physiology

Accelerations in fetal heart rate occur in association with fetal movement, probably as a result of stimulation of peripheral proprioceptors, increased catecholamine release, and autonomic stimulation of the heart. In the third trimester, spontaneous accelerations occur at a rate of 10 to 20 per hour. In the absence of spontaneous accelerations, fetal scalp stimulation or vibroacoustic stimulation can provoke fetal movement and fetal heart rate accelerations.

Interpretation

Fetal oxygenation: Accelerations, like moderate variability, reflect normal autonomic regulation of the fetal heart rate. The presence of accelerations indicates that autonomic regulation of the fetal heart rate is not blunted by disrupted oxygenation that has progressed to the stage of metabolic acidemia. *A central concept of electronic fetal heart rate monitoring is that fetal heart rate accelerations are highly predictive of the absence of fetal metabolic acidemia.*[9,11,35,42] Supporting evidence is Levels II-2, II-3, and III.

Other mechanisms: Accelerations indicate that autonomic regulation of the fetal heart rate is not significantly affected by fetal sleep, tachycardia, prematurity, congenital anomalies, central nervous system depressants, or medications.[14,16,24,47] Another suspected mechanism of fetal heart rate acceleration is transient compression of the umbilical vein, resulting in decreased fetal venous return and a reflex rise in heart rate. Evidence is Level III.

DECELERATIONS

Definition

Fetal heart rate decelerations are categorized as late, early, variable, or prolonged. Late decelerations and early decelerations are gradual in onset and periodic in timing (associated with uterine contractions). Variable decelerations are abrupt in onset and may be periodic or episodic (unrelated to contractions). Prolonged decelerations may be abrupt or gradual in onset and may be periodic or episodic in timing. Decelerations are defined as recurrent if they occur with at least 50% of uterine contractions in any 20-minute segment. All decelerations may be quantitated by depth in beats per minute below the baseline (excluding transient spikes or electronic artifact) and duration in minutes and seconds from the beginning to the end of the deceleration. Standardized NICHD terminology does not classify fetal heart rate decelerations as "mild," "moderate," or "severe." The following sections review the standard definition and interpretation of each pattern.

Physiology

Decelerations in the fetal heart rate are caused by two basic physiologic mechanisms:

1. Reflex autonomic slowing of the FHR in response to changes in blood pressure, blood gases, and possibly other factors
2. Direct depression of the FHR resulting from disrupted oxygenation of the myocardium

The first mechanism is responsible for the majority of fetal heart rate decelerations encountered in clinical practice. The second mechanism is much less common, but may come into play after a period of recurrent or sustained disruption of fetal oxygenation. Scientific evidence supporting these mechanisms ranges from Level II-1 to Level III.

LATE DECELERATIONS

Definition

Late deceleration of the fetal heart rate is defined as a gradual (onset to nadir ≥30 seconds) decrease of the fetal heart rate from the baseline and subsequent return to the baseline associated with a uterine contraction (Figure 5-12). The decrease is calculated from the most recently determined portion of the baseline. In most cases the onset, nadir, and recovery of the deceleration occur after the beginning, peak, and ending of the contraction, respectively. Late decelerations are defined as recurrent if they occur with at least 50% of uterine contractions in any 20-minute segment.

Interpretation

Fetal oxygenation: A late deceleration is a reflex fetal response to transient hypoxemia during a uterine contraction. Myometrial contractions can compress maternal blood vessels traversing the uterine wall and disrupt maternal perfusion of the intervillous space of the placenta. Reduced delivery of oxygenated blood to the intervillous space can reduce the diffusion of oxygen into the fetal capillary blood in the chorionic villi, leading to a decline in fetal Po_2 below the normal range of approximately 15 to 25 mm Hg. If the fetal Po_2 falls below a critical threshold, chemoreceptors detect the change and signal medullary vasomotor centers to initiate a protective reflex response. Sympathetic outflow causes peripheral vasoconstriction and centralization

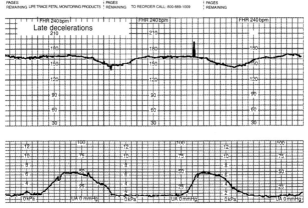

FIGURE 5-12 Late decelerations.

of blood volume, favoring perfusion of the brain, heart, and adrenal glands. The resulting increase in peripheral resistance causes a rise in mean arterial blood pressure and a subsequent baroreceptor-mediated reflex slowing of the heart rate to reduce cardiac output and return the blood pressure to normal. This mechanism has been elucidated elegantly in a number of animal studies,* and it is summarized in Figure 5-13.

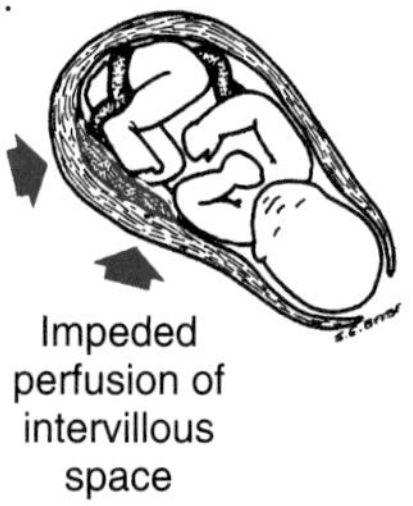

Impeded
perfusion of
intervillous
space

Physiologic mechanism of late deceleration

Uterine contraction impedes
maternal perfusion of the
placental intervillous space
↓
Transient fetal hypoxemia ⟶
↓
Chemoreceptor stimulation
↓
Reflex sympathetic outflow
↓
Peripheral vasoconstriction, preferentially
shunting oxygenated blood away from the
peripheral tissues and toward central vital
organs: brain, heart, adrenal glands
↓
Increase in fetal peripheral resistance
and blood pressure
↓
Baroreceptor stimulation
↓
Reflex parasympathetic outflow
↓
Gradual slowing of the FHR
↓
Late deceleration ⟵
↓
After the contraction, these reflexes subside

Note: In the presence
of fetal metabolic
acidemia, transient
hypoxemia may result
in myocardial
hypoxia and a late
deceleration secondary
to direct
myocardial depression

FIGURE 5-13 Physiologic mechanism of late deceleration.

*References 5,6,10,12,21,23,29,34,36,37

If disruption of fetal oxygenation is recurrent or sustained, it may progress to the stage of metabolic acidemia. In the setting of metabolic acidemia, a late deceleration can reflect a direct myocardial depressant effect of hypoxia. In that event, other fetal heart rate abnormalities would be expected, such as fetal tachycardia, absent variability, and absent accelerations.

For the purpose of standardized interpretation of intrapartum fetal heart rate patterns, a late deceleration reflects transient disruption of oxygen transfer from the environment to the fetus resulting in transient fetal hypoxemia. The scientific evidence supporting the physiologic basis of a late deceleration is Level II-1 and Level II-2.

Other mechanisms: No other mechanisms are known to cause late decelerations.

EARLY DECELERATIONS

Definition

Early deceleration is defined as a gradual (onset to nadir ≥30 seconds) decrease in fetal heart rate from the baseline and subsequent return to baseline associated with a uterine contraction (Figure 5-14). In most cases the onset, nadir, and recovery of the deceleration occur at the same time as the beginning, peak, and end of the contraction, respectively. Early decelerations are defined as recurrent if they occur with at least 50% of uterine contractions in any 20-minute segment.

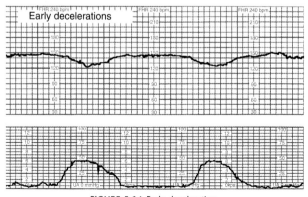

FIGURE 5-14 Early deceleration.

Interpretation

Fetal oxygenation: Early decelerations have no known relationship to fetal oxygenation.

Other mechanisms: The presumed physiologic mechanism of early deceleration is depicted in Figure 5-15. Although the precise physiologic mechanism is not known, early decelerations are thought to represent a fetal autonomic response to changes in intracranial pressure and/or cerebral blood flow caused by intrapartum compression of the fetal head.

These decelerations do not appear to be associated with poor outcome and, therefore, are considered clinically benign. Evidence is Level II-3 and Level III.

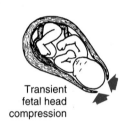

Transient
fetal head
compression

Physiologic mechanism of early deceleration

Transient fetal head compression
↓
Altered intracranial pressure and/or cerebral blood flow
↓
Reflex parasympathetic outflow
↓
Gradual slowing of the FHR
↓
Early deceleration
↓
When head compression is relieved, autonomic reflexes subside

FIGURE 5-15 Physiologic mechanism of early deceleration.

VARIABLE DECELERATIONS

Definition

Variable deceleration of the fetal heart rate is defined as an abrupt (onset to nadir <30 seconds) decrease in fetal heart rate below the baseline, calculated from the most recently determined portion of the baseline (Figure 5-16). The decrease in fetal heart rate below the baseline is at least 15 beats per minute and the deceleration lasts at least 15 seconds and less than 2 minutes from onset to return to baseline. Variable decelerations are not necessarily associated with uterine contractions. However, when they are, the onset, depth, and duration commonly vary with successive uterine contractions. In addition, if they are associated with uterine contractions, variable decelerations are defined as recurrent if they occur with at least 50% of uterine contractions in any 20-minute segment.

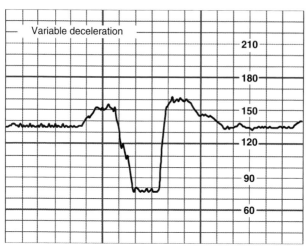

FIGURE 5-16 Variable deceleration.

Interpretation

Fetal oxygenation: Variable decelerations result from transient mechanical compression of umbilical blood vessels within the umbilical cord.* Initially, compression of the umbilical cord

---

*References 7,19,20,22,26,27,30,41,44,48

occludes the thin-walled, compliant umbilical vein, decreasing fetal venous return and triggering a baroreceptor-mediated reflex rise in fetal heart rate (commonly described as a "shoulder"). Further compression of the umbilical cord results in occlusion of the umbilical arteries, causing an abrupt increase in fetal peripheral resistance and blood pressure. Baroreceptors detect the abrupt rise in blood pressure and signal the medullary vasomotor center which, in turn, triggers an increase in parasympathetic outflow along the vagus nerve and an abrupt decrease in heart rate. Parasympathetic stimulation of the heart may result in a junctional or idioventricular rhythm that appears as a relatively stable rate of

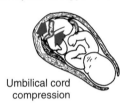

Umbilical cord
compression

Physiologic mechanism of variable deceleration

Umbilical cord compression
↓
Initial compression of umbilical vein
↓
Transient decreased fetal venous return
↓
Transient reduction in fetal cardiac output and blood pressure
↓
Baroreceptor stimulation
↓
Transient reflex rise in FHR
↓
Umbilical artery compression
↓
Abrupt rise in fetal peripheral resistance and blood pressure
↓
Baroreceptor stimulation
↓
Reflex parasympathetic outflow
↓
Abrupt slowing of the FHR
↓
Variable deceleration
↓
When umbilical cord compression is relieved, this process occurs in reverse

FIGURE 5-17 Physiologic mechanism of variable deceleration.

60 to 80 beats per minute at the base of a variable deceleration. As the cord is decompressed, this sequence of events occurs in reverse.

A shoulder is also common following a variable deceleration. It is important to note that the term *shoulder* is not included in the standard NICHD definitions of fetal heart rate patterns. This term, and others lacking standard definitions, is addressed in a separate section of this chapter. Umbilical cord compression results in transient disruption of normal oxygen transfer from the environment to the fetus. During a variable deceleration, the fetal P_{O_2} may or may not fall below the normal range of 15 to 25 mm Hg. Regardless of the impact on fetal P_{O_2}, a variable deceleration is transient by definition (duration <2 min), and occasional compression of the umbilical cord usually has little clinical significance. Recurrent variable decelerations, on the other hand, can result in recurrent disruption of fetal oxygenation and lead to a cascade of progressive physiologic changes including hypoxemia, hypoxia, metabolic acidosis, and eventually metabolic acidemia. In that event, associated fetal heart rate observations may include a rising baseline rate, minimal or absent variability, absent accelerations, and slow return to baseline following decelerations. The last of these has been referred to as a *variable with a late component.* This term is not defined by the NICHD and is addressed later in the chapter.

For the purpose of fetal heart rate interpretation, a variable deceleration reflects transient disruption of oxygen transfer from the environment to the fetus at the level of the umbilical cord. The physiologic mechanism of variable deceleration is depicted in Figure 5-17. Supporting evidence is Levels II-1, II-2, II-3, and III.

Other mechanisms: Another suggested physiologic mechanism resulting in variable deceleration is a fetal vagal response to umbilical cord stretching. This mechanism may be similar to the mechanism underlying umbilical cord compression. Supporting evidence is limited (Level III).

PROLONGED DECELERATIONS

Definition

Prolonged deceleration of the fetal heart rate is defined as a decrease (either gradual or abrupt) in fetal heart rate of at least 15 beats per

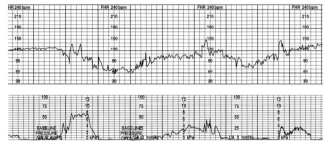

FIGURE 5-18 Prolonged decelerations.

minute below the baseline lasting at least 2 minutes from onset to return to baseline (Figure 5-18). According to NICHD terminology, a prolonged deceleration lasting 10 minutes or longer is defined as a baseline change. Under no circumstances should this statement be interpreted to suggest that a prolonged deceleration turns into a benign baseline change after 10 minutes.

Interpretation

Fetal oxygenation: A prolonged deceleration reflects disrupted oxygen transfer from the environment to the fetus at one or more points along the oxygen pathway. As described in the introduction to fetal heart rate decelerations, there are two basic physiologic mechanisms:

1. Reflex autonomic response
2. Direct myocardial depression

A prolonged deceleration usually begins as a reflex autonomic response to disruption of the oxygen pathway. If the oxygen pathway is disrupted by mechanical compression of the umbilical cord, the fetal heart rate deceleration begins as a reflex autonomic response to fetal hypertension. Alternatively, an acute event such as placental abruption or uterine rupture can cause an abrupt fall in fetal P_{O_2}. Reflex peripheral vasoconstriction centralizes blood volume and increases blood pressure. The resulting fetal heart rate deceleration begins as a reflex autonomic response to the rise in blood pressure triggered by falling P_{O_2}. Regardless of the cause, sustained disruption of oxygen transfer can lead to progressive physiologic changes, including fetal hypoxemia, hypoxia, metabolic acidosis, and metabolic acidemia. Eventually, tissue hypoxia and acidosis can lead to failure of peripheral vascular smooth muscle contraction. The resultant fetal hypotension reduces diastolic blood pressure and compromises coronary blood flow, leading to myocardial hypoxia, direct myocardial depression, and slowing of the fetal heart rate. If this process is not corrected, the heart may stop beating altogether. It is likely that both mechanisms (autonomic reflex and direct myocardial depression) contribute to the underlying physiology of a prolonged fetal heart rate deceleration; however, their precise relative roles are not known. In general, autonomic reflexes appear to predominate initially, and hypoxic myocardial depression appears to be a later mechanism.

For the purpose of fetal heart rate interpretation, a prolonged deceleration reflects disruption of oxygen transfer from the environment to the fetus at one or more points along the oxygen pathway. Supporting evidence is Levels II-1, II-2, II-3, and III.

Other mechanisms: Other proposed mechanisms of prolonged decelerations can overlap with those causing fetal bradycardia. Examples include fetal heart failure, maternal hypoglycemia, and hypothermia. Supporting evidence is Level III.

PATTERNS NOT DEFINED BY THE NATIONAL INSTITUTE OF CHILD HEALTH AND HUMAN DEVELOPMENT

Several terms that were not defined in the NICHD report are common in clinical practice. Some of these are discussed below.

"Wandering Baseline"

A fetal heart rate baseline that is within the normal range (110-160 beats per minute) but is not stable at a single rate for long enough to define a mean has been described as a "wandering baseline." Absent variability and absent accelerations are prominent features (Figure 5-19). Decelerations can be present or absent. This combination of fetal heart rate findings has been suggested to indicate preexisting neurologic injury and impending fetal death. The physiologic mechanism is not known and published data are limited (Level III). If this pattern is observed, it should be interpreted in the context of other fetal heart rate observations and clinical factors.

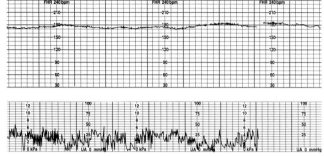

FIGURE 5-19 Wandering baseline.

"Lambda" Pattern

The lambda fetal heart rate pattern (Figure 5-20) is characterized by a brief acceleration followed by a small deceleration.[8] Common during early labor, this pattern has no known clinical significance. The underlying physiologic mechanism is not known (Level III).

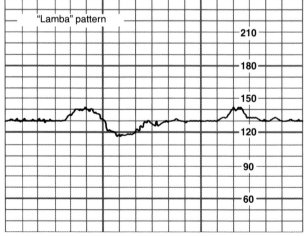

FIGURE 5-20 Lambda pattern.

"Shoulder(s)"

As discussed above, variable decelerations result from transient mechanical compression of umbilical blood vessels within the umbilical cord. Initial compression of the umbilical vein reduces fetal venous return and triggers a baroreceptor-mediated reflex rise in fetal heart rate that commonly is described as a "shoulder"[22,27] (Figure 5-21). As the cord is decompressed, a second shoulder frequently follows the deceleration and likely reflects the same underlying mechanism. The precise mechanism has not been confirmed, but there is little reason to suspect that the above explanation is substantially inaccurate. There is no known association with adverse newborn outcome. On the other hand, there is no firm evidence that the observation reflects normal fetal oxygenation. It is considered a clinically benign observation. Supporting evidence is Level III.

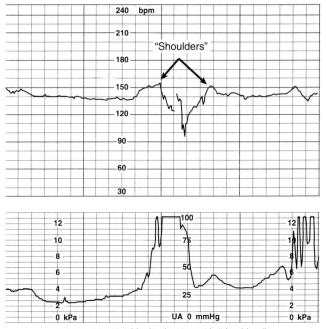

FIGURE 5-21 Variable deceleration with "shoulders."

"Checkmark" Pattern

The checkmark pattern is an unusual fetal heart rate pattern that has been described in association with neurologic injury, neonatal convulsions, and possible in utero fetal seizure activity. It is depicted in Figure 5-22. Unlike most fetal heart rate patterns described in association with neurologic injury, the checkmark pattern is not necessarily accompanied by absent baseline variability. All evidence related to the visual appearance of the pattern and the putative clinical significance is Level III.

"End-Stage" Bradycardia and "Terminal" Bradycardia

Standardized NICHD fetal heart rate terminology clearly indicates that the term bradycardia applies to the baseline fetal heart rate. The term specifically does not apply to a prolonged deceleration that interrupts the baseline. The terms "end-stage" bradycardia and "terminal" bradycardia have been used to describe a prolonged deceleration observed at the end of the second stage of labor (Figure 5-23). Such decelerations are common in the course of normal vaginal delivery and usually are of little clinical significance.

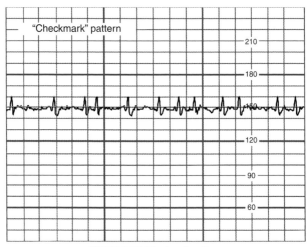

FIGURE 5-22 Checkmark pattern.

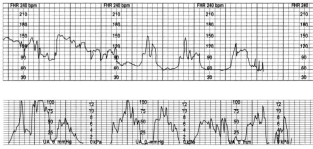

FIGURE 5-23 End-stage or terminal bradycardia. Note the more precise term would be *prolonged decelerations*.

The precise cause is unknown; however, suggested mechanisms include umbilical cord compression, umbilical cord stretching, fetal head compression, and transient fetal hypoxemia due to excessive uterine activity and/or maternal expulsive efforts. The impact on immediate newborn outcome is variable and depends upon a number of interacting factors, including, but not limited to, the physiologic cause of the deceleration, prior condition of the fetus, and duration of the deceleration. Consistent with NICHD terminology, the terms *end-stage bradycardia* and *terminal bradycardia* should be discarded in favor of the more precise term *prolonged decelerations*. Evidence is Level III.

"Uniform" Accelerations

Various terms have been used to describe fetal heart rate accelerations associated with uterine contractions, including "uniform sporadic accelerations", "variable sporadic accelerations", "uniform periodic accelerations", "sporadic periodic accelerations", and "crown accelerations". These terms are not included in standardized NICHD definitions, and there is no documented physiologic basis for such subclassification.

"Atypical" Variable Decelerations

"Overshoot"

The term "overshoot" has been used to describe a fetal heart rate pattern characterized by persistently absent variability, absent accelerations, and a variable deceleration followed by a smooth, prolonged rise in the fetal heart rate above the previous baseline with gradual return[15,38-40,46] (Figure 5-24). As with the wandering baseline, essential elements of this uncommon pattern include the persistent absence of variability and the absence of accelerations.

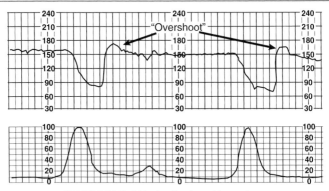

FIGURE 5-24 Variable deceleration with overshoot.

The overshoot pattern has been attributed to a range of conditions, including mild fetal hypoxia above the deceleration threshold, chronic fetal distress, and repetitive transient central nervous system ischemia. However, all of these associations are speculative and none has been substantiated by available scientific evidence. The physiologic mechanisms responsible for the overshoot pattern are not known. However, the pattern has been described in association with abnormal neurologic outcome with or without metabolic acidemia, suggesting that it might indicate preexisting neurologic injury. Because of the wide variation in reported associations and the lack of agreement regarding the definition and clinical significance of *overshoot,* it is best to avoid the use of this term in favor of more specific terminology. All evidence regarding the overshoot pattern in humans is Level III.

"Variable Deceleration With a Late Component"

The phrase "variable deceleration with a late component" has been used to describe a deceleration with an abrupt onset and a gradual return to baseline, as seen in Figure 5-25. The abrupt onset suggests that the deceleration begins as a reflex autonomic response to an abrupt rise in blood pressure caused by umbilical cord compression (the "variable" component of the pattern). The gradual return to baseline suggests a gradual reduction of autonomic outflow upon resolution of transient hypoxemia, as occurs in a late deceleration (the "late" component of the pattern). A plausible explanation of the pattern would be initial umbilical cord compression causing a reflex fall in fetal heart rate and a transient decline in fetal Po_2. The Po_2 probably drops below the threshold that triggers the reflex sympathetic outflow and peripheral vasoconstriction characteristic

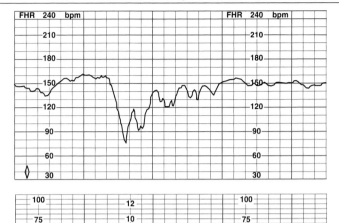

FIGURE 5-25 Variable deceleration with late component.

of a late deceleration. Decompression of the umbilical cord brings about rapid resolution of the variable deceleration; however, the physiologic mechanisms responsible for late deceleration resolve more slowly, causing the fetal heart rate to return slowly to the previous baseline. Although the specific physiologic mechanism has not been studied systematically, this explanation is a reasonable extrapolation from known mechanisms.

Scientific evidence regarding the underlying physiologic mechanism is limited to Level III. Second-stage variable decelerations with slow recovery have been reported to increase the likelihood of operative delivery; however, no consistent impact on newborn outcome has been described.[43] In the absence of a standard definition of this pattern, its use is best avoided in favor of standard terminology with additional descriptors, for example, "variable deceleration with gradual return to baseline."

"Mild", "Moderate", and "Severe" Variable Decelerations

The depth and duration of variable decelerations have been suggested as predictors of newborn outcome. Kubli and colleagues proposed three categories of variable decelerations based upon these characteristics.[25] According to this classification system, a mild variable deceleration was defined by a duration less than 30 seconds regardless of depth, a depth no lower than 80 beats per minute, or a depth of 70 to 80 beats per minute lasting less than 60 seconds. A moderate variable deceleration was defined by a depth less than 70 beats per minute lasting 30 to 60 seconds or a depth of 70 to 80 beats per minute lasting more than 60 seconds. A severe deceleration was defined as a deceleration below 70 beats per minute lasting more than 60 seconds.

There is no conclusive evidence in the literature that the depth of any type of deceleration (early, variable, late, or prolonged) is predictive of fetal metabolic acidemia or newborn outcome *independent* of other important fetal heart rate characteristics such as baseline rate, variability, accelerations, and frequency of decelerations. Therefore, mild, moderate, and severe categories are not included in standard NICHD definitions of fetal heart rate decelerations. Consistent with NICHD terminology, all decelerations may be further quantitated by depth in beats per minute and duration in minutes and seconds. For further discussion on quantification of decelerations, see Chapter 10.

"V-shaped" and "W-shaped" Variables

The visual appearance of a variable deceleration has been suggested to predict the underlying cause. For example, a "V-shaped" variable deceleration has been suggested to indicate umbilical cord compression due to oligohydramnios, while a "W-shaped" variable deceleration has been suggested to reflect umbilical cord compression due to a nuchal cord (Figure 5-26). Although such claims likely have little impact on patient care, there is no supporting evidence in the literature. These terms are not included in standardized NICHD terminology.

"Good Variability Within the Deceleration"

At the nadir of a variable or late deceleration, the fetal heart rate frequently appears irregular, similar to the appearance of moderate variability. The visual similarity has led some to suggest that variability during a deceleration has the same clinical significance as baseline variability. Although the concept is physiologically plausible, it has never been studied. In addition, it is inconsistent with

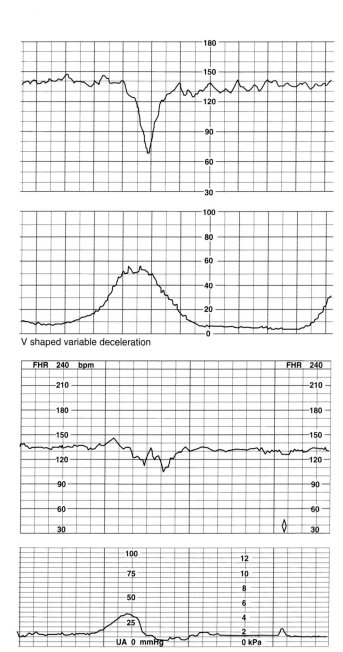

V shaped variable deceleration

W shaped variable deceleration

FIGURE 5-26 V-shaped versus W-shaped variable decelerations.

standard terminology. Variability is a characteristic of the fetal heart rate baseline. The term *variability* is not used to qualify periodic or episodic decelerations that interrupt the baseline. In the absence of evidence, the safest approach is to avoid assigning undue significance to this observation.

SUMMARY

The three basic elements of fetal heart rate monitoring are (1) terminology, (2) interpretation, and (3) management. A standardized, evidence-based approach to each element facilitates effective communication, promotes patient safety, and helps ensure optimal outcomes.

Standardized terminology has been endorsed by all major professional organizations in the United States representing providers of obstetric care. The simple agreement to adopt a common language sets the stage for the next essential step. Standardized fetal heart rate interpretation requires a critical assessment of the scientific evidence underlying the relationships between fetal heart rate patterns and fetal physiology.

As described in Chapter 2, the physiologic basis of fetal heart rate monitoring can be summarized in some key concepts, outlined below.

- The objective of intrapartum FHR monitoring is to assess fetal oxygenation.
- Fetal oxygenation involves the transfer of oxygen from the environment to the fetus and the subsequent fetal response.
- Transfer of oxygen from the environment to the fetus follows a common pathway that invariably includes the maternal lungs, heart, vasculature, uterus, placenta, and umbilical cord.
- Fetal response to disrupted oxygen transfer involves the sequential physiologic progression from hypoxemia to hypoxia, metabolic acidosis, metabolic acidemia, and finally, hypotension.
- Fetal neurologic injury due to disrupted oxygenation does not occur unless it has progressed at least to the stage of significant metabolic acidemia (umbilical artery pH < 7.0 and base deficit ≥ 12 mmol/L).

This chapter has reviewed in detail the relationships between specific fetal heart rate patterns and fetal physiology with particular emphasis on evidence-based interpretation. Regarding the relationship between fetal heart rate patterns and fetal oxygenation, evidence-based fetal heart rate interpretation can be distilled into three basic statements:

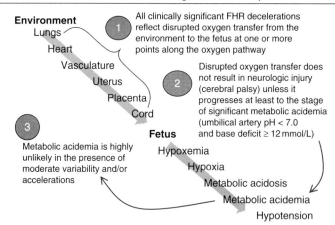

Environment
Lungs
Heart
Vasculature
Uterus
Placenta
Cord
Fetus
Hypoxemia
Hypoxia
Metabolic acidosis
Metabolic acidemia
Hypotension

① All clinically significant FHR decelerations reflect disrupted oxygen transfer from the environment to the fetus at one or more points along the oxygen pathway

② Disrupted oxygen transfer does not result in neurologic injury (cerebral palsy) unless it progresses at least to the stage of significant metabolic acidemia (umbilical artery pH < 7.0 and base deficit ≥ 12 mmol/L)

③ Metabolic acidemia is highly unlikely in the presence of moderate variability and/or accelerations

FIGURE 5-27 Intrapartum FHR monitoring interpretation. (Courtesy David A. Miller, MD.)

1. All clinically significant FHR decelerations reflect disruption of oxygen transfer from the environment to the fetus at one or more points along the oxygen pathway.
2. Fetal neurologic injury due to disrupted oxygen transfer does not occur unless it progresses at least to the stage of significant metabolic acidemia (umbilical artery pH<7.0 and base deficit 12 mmol/L).[3]
3. Significant metabolic acidemia is highly unlikely in the presence of moderate FHR variability and/or accelerations.

These concepts, illustrated in Figure 5-27, form the basis of systematic management of fetal heart rate patterns discussed in Chapter 6.

References

1. American College of Nurse-Midwives: *Standard nomenclature for electronic fetal monitoring, Position Statement 2006*, Silver Spring, MD, 2006, ACNM.
2. American College of Obstetricians and Gynecologists: Intrapartum fetal heart rate monitoring, ACOG *Practice Bulletin* no.70, *Obstet Gynecol* 106(6):1453-1461, 2005.
3. American College of Obstetricians and Gynecologists Task Force on Neonatal Encephalopathy and Cerebral Palsy, American College of Obstetricians and Gynecologists, American Academy of Pediatrics: *Neonatal encephalopathy and cerebral palsy: Defining the pathogenesis and pathophysiology*, Washington, 2003, ACOG, AAP.

4. Association of Women's Health, Obstetric and Neonatal Nurses: *Changes to the FHMPP program.* Accessed August 22, 2005, from www.awhonn.org/awhonn/?pg=873-2180-17530.

5. Ball RH, Espinoza MI, Parer JT: Regional blood flow in asphyxiated fetuses with seizures, *Am J Obstet Gynecol* 170(1 Pt 1):156-261, 1994.

6. Ball RH, Parer JT, Caldwell LE, Johnson J: Regional blood flow and metabolism ovine fetuses during severe cord occlusion, *Am J Obstet Gynecol* 171(6):1549-1555, 1994.

7. Barcroft J: *Researches in prenatal life,* Oxford, 1946, Blackwell.

8. Brubaker K, Garite TJ: The lambda fetal heart rate pattern: An assessment of its significance in the intrapartum period, *Obstet Gynecol* 72 (6):881-885, 1988.

9. Clark SL, Gimovski ML, Miller FC: Fetal heart rate response to scalp blood sampling, *Am J Obstet Gynecol* 144(6):706-708, 1982.

10. Cohn HE, Sacks EJ, Heymann MA, Rudolph AM: Cardiovascular response to hypoxemia and acidemia in fetal lambs, *Am J Obstet Gynecol* 120(6):817-824, 1974.

11. Elimian A, Figueroa R, Tejani N: Intrapartum assessment of fetal well being: A comparison of scalp stimulation with scalp blood pH sampling, *Obstet Gynecol* 89(3):373-376, 1997.

12. Field DR, Parer JT, Auslander RA, Cheek DB, Baker W, Johnson J: Cerebral oxygen consumption during asphyxia in fetal sheep, *J Dev Physiol* 14(3):131-137, 1990.

13. Fleischer, A, Schulman, H, Jagani, N, Mitchell, J and Randolph G: The development of fetal acidosis in the presence of an abnormal fetal heart rate tracing. I. The average for gestational age fetus, *Am J Obstet Gynecol* 144(1):55-60, 1982.

14. Giannina G, Guzman ER, Lai YL, Lake MF, Cernadas M, Vintzileos AM: Comparison of the effects of meperidine and nalbuphine on intrapartum fetal heart rate tracings, *Obstet Gynecol* 86(3):441-445, 1995.

15. Goodlin RC, Lowe EW: A functional umbilical cord occlusion heart rate pattern. The significance of overshoot, *Obstet Gynecol* 43(1):22-30, 1974.

16. Hallak M, Martinez-Poyer J, Kruger ML, Hassan S, Blackwell SC, Sorokin Y: The effect of magnesium sulfate on fetal heart rate parameters: A randomized, placebo-controlled trial, *Am J Obstet Gynecol* 181(5 Pt 1):1122-1127, 1999.

17. Hatjis CG, Meis PJ: Sinusoidal fetal heart rate pattern associated with butorphanol administration, *Obstet Gynecol* 67(3):377-380, 1986.

18. Ingemarsson I, Herbst A, Thorgren-Jerneck K: Long-term outcome after umbilical artery acidemia at term birth: Influence of gender and fetal heart rate abnormalities, *Br J Obstet Gynaecol* 104(10):1123-1127, 1997.

19. Itskovitz J, LaGamma EF, Rudolph AM: The effect of reducing umbilical blood flow on fetal oxygenation, *Am J Obstet Gynecol* 145(7):813-818, 1983.

20. Itskovitz J, LaGamma EF, Rudolph AM: Heart rate and blood pressure responses to umbilical cord compression in fetal lambs with special

reference to the mechanism of variable deceleration, *Am J Obstet Gynecol* 147(4):451-457, 1983.

21. Itskovitz J, LaGamma EF, Rudolph AM: Effect of cord compression on fetal blood flow distribution and O_2 delivery, *Am J Physiol* 252(1 Pt 2): H100-H109, 1987.

22. James LS, Yeh MN, Morishima HO, Daniel SS, Caritis SN, Niemann WH, Indyk L: Umbilical vein occlusion and transient acceleration of the fetal heart rate. Experimental observations in subhuman primates, *Am J Obstet Gynecol* 126(2):276-283, 1976.

23. Jensen A, Roman C, Rudolph A:. Effects of reducing uterine blood flow on fetal blood flow distribution and oxygen delivery, *J Dev Physiol* 15 (6):309-323, 1991.

24. Kopecky EA, Ryan ML, Barrett JF, Seaward PG, Ryan G, Koren G, Amankwah K: Fetal response to maternally administered morphine, *Am J Obstet Gynecol* 183(2):424-430, 2000.

25. Kubli FW, Hon EH, Khazin AF, Takemura H: Observations on heart rate and pH in the human fetus during labor, *Am J Obstet Gynecol* 104 (8):1190-1206, 1969.

26. Lee CY, Di Loreto PC, O'Lane JM: A study of fetal heart rate acceleration patterns, *Obstet Gynecol* 45(2):142-146, 1975.

27. Lee ST, Hon EH: Fetal hemodynamic response to umbilical cord compression, *Obstet Gynecol* 22:553-562, 1963.

28. Low JA, Galbraith RS, Muir DW, Killen HL, Pater EA, Karchmar EJ: Factors associated with motor and cognitive deficits in children after intrapartum fetal hypoxia, *Am J Obstet Gynecol* 148:533-539, 1982.

29. Martin CB Jr, de Haan J, van der Wildt B, Jongsma HW, Dieleman A, Arts TH: Mechanisms of late decelerations in the fetal heart rate. A study with autonomic blocking agents in fetal lambs, *Eur J Obstet Gynecol Reprod Biol* 9(6):361-373, 1979.

30. Mueller-Heubach E, Battelli AF: Variable heart rate decelerations and transcutaneous Po_2 during umbilical cord occlusion in fetal monkeys, *Am J Obstet Gynecol* 144(7):796-802, 1982.

31. National Institute of Child Health and Human Development Research Planning Workshop: Electronic fetal heart rate monitoring: Research guidelines for interpretation, *Am J Obstet Gynecol* 177(6):1385-1390, 1997.

32. Parer JT, Ikeda T: A framework for standardized management of intrapartum fetal heart rate patterns, *Am J Obstet Gynecol* 197(1):26e1-e6, 2007.

33. Parer JT, King T, Flanders S, Fox M, Kilpatrick SJ: Fetal acidemia and electronic fetal heart rate patterns: Is there evidence of an association? *J Matern Fetal Neonatal Med* 19(5):289-294, 2006.

34. Peeters LL, Sheldon RD, Jones MD, Makowski EL, Meschia G: Blood flow to fetal organs as a function of arterial oxygen content, *Am J Obstet Gynecol* 135(5):637-646, 1979.

35. Read JA, Miller FC: Fetal heart rate acceleration in response to acoustic stimulation as a measure of fetal well-being, *Am J Obstet Gynecol* 129 (5):512-517, 1977.

36. Reid DL, Parer JT, Williams K, Darr D, Phermaton TM, Rankin JHH: Effects of severe reduction in maternal placental blood flow on blood flow distribution in the sheep fetus, *J Dev Physiol* 15(3):183-188, 1991.

37. Richardson BS, Rurak D, Patrick JE, Homan J, Carmichael L: Cerebral oxidative metabolism during prolonged hypoxemia, *J Dev Physiol* 11 (1):37-43, 1989.

38. Saito J, Okamura K, Akagi K, Tanigawara S, Shintaku Y, Watanabe T, Akiyama N, Endo C, Sato A, Yajima A: Alteration of FHR pattern associated with progressively advanced fetal acidemia caused by cord compression, *Nippon Sanka Fujinka Gakkai Zasshi* 40(6):775-780, 1988.

39. Schifrin BS, Hamilton-Rubinstein T, Shield JR: Fetal heart rate patterns and the timing of fetal injury, *J Perinatol* 14(3):174-181, 1994.

40. Shields JR, Schifrin BS: Perinatal antecedents of cerebral palsy. *Obstet Gynecol* 71(6 Pt 1):899-905, 1988.

41. Siassi B, Wu, PY, Blanco C, Martin CB: Baroreceptor and chemoreceptor responses to umbilical cord occlusion in fetal lambs, *Biol Neonate* 35 (1-2):66-73, 1979.

42. Smith CV, Nguyen HN, Phelan JP, Paul RH: Intrapartum assessment of fetal well-being: A comparison of fetal acoustic stimulation with acid base determinations, *Am J Obstet Gynecol* 155(4):726-728, 1986.

43. Spong CY, Rascul C, Collea JY, Eglinton GS, Ghidini A: Characterization and prognostic significance of variable decelerations in the second stage of labor, *Am J Perinatol* 15(6):369-374, 1998.

44. Towell MD, Salvador HS: Compression of the umbilical cord. In Crasignoni P, Pardi G, editors: *An experimental model in the fetal goat, fetal evaluation during pregnancy and labor*, pp. 143-156, New York, 1971, Academic Press.

45. U.S. Preventive Services Task Force: *Guide to Clinical Preventative Services. Report of the U.S. Preventive Services Task Force*, ed 2, Philadelphia, 1996, Lippincott Williams and Wilkins.

46. Westgate JA, Bennet L, de Haan HH, Gunn AJ: Fetal heart rate overshoot during repeated umbilical cord occlusion in sheep, *Obstet Gynecol* 97(3):454-459, 2001.

47. Wright JW, Ridgway LE, Wright BD, Covington DL, Bobitt JR: Effect of MgSO4 on heart rate monitoring in the preterm fetus, *J Reprod Med* 41(8):605-608, 1996.

48. Yeh MN, Morishima HO, Niemann WE, James LS: Myocardial conduction defects in association with compression of the umbilical cord. Experimental observations on fetal baboons, *Am J Obstet Gynecol* 121 (7):951-957, 1975.

CHAPTER 6

Management of the Intrapartum Fetal Heart Rate Tracing

The physiologic basis for fetal heart rate (FHR) monitoring and evaluation of uterine activity were reviewed in Chapters 2 and 4. Standardized National Institute of Child Health and Human Development (NICHD) terminology and evidence-based interpretation of fetal heart rate patterns were presented in Chapter 5. This chapter incorporates the concepts developed previously and presents a systematic, comprehensive approach to the decision-making process underlying the management of intrapartum fetal heart rate tracings. As emphasized previously, fetal heart rate patterns do not occur alone and generally evolve over time. Effective management addresses all five essential components of a fetal heart rate tracing together: (1) baseline rate, (2) baseline variability, (3) accelerations, (4) presence or absence of decelerations, and (5) changes or trends in the tracing over time. *Emphasis is placed on the primary objective of intrapartum fetal heart rate monitoring: to prevent fetal injury that might result from disrupted fetal oxygenation during labor.*

MANAGEMENT

General Considerations

Reliable information is vital to the success of intrapartum fetal heart rate monitoring. Therefore, it is essential to confirm that the monitor is recording the fetal heart rate and uterine activity accurately and that the tracing in interpretable. Ultrasound might be necessary to locate the fetal heart rate or to confirm that the observed rate is fetal and not maternal. If external monitoring is not adequate for interpretation, a fetal scalp electrode and/or intrauterine pressure catheter might be necessary.

Fundamental Principles

As introduced at the close of Chapter 5, there are *three central concepts of evidence-based fetal heart rate interpretation.* These concepts provide the foundation for a systematic approach to the decision-making process underlying fetal heart rate management. They are as follows:

1. All clinically significant FHR decelerations reflect disruption of oxygen transfer from the environment to the fetus at one or more points along the oxygen pathway.

2. Fetal neurologic injury due to disrupted oxygen transfer does not occur unless it progresses at least to the stage of significant metabolic acidemia (umbilical artery pH <7.0 and base deficit ≥12 mmol/L).[8]

3. Significant metabolic acidemia is highly unlikely in the presence of moderate FHR variability and/or accelerations.

Figure 6-1 illustrates the relationship of these three concepts to both the oxygen pathway and the fetal response to hypoxia.

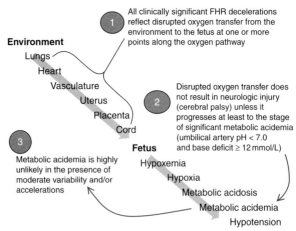

FIGURE 6-1 Three central concepts of FHR interpretation. (Courtesy David A. Miller, MD.)

EVALUATE THE FETAL HEART RATE TRACING

After confirming that the monitor is accurately and adequately recording the necessary information, the fetal heart rate tracing is evaluated. Two initial issues are addressed:

1. Does the FHR tracing mandate immediate intervention (e.g., a prolonged deceleration that does not recover despite corrective measures)? If so, immediate action should be taken to expedite delivery.
2. Are there are other indications to expedite delivery (e.g., bleeding placenta previa or severe preeclampsia)? If so, management is determined by the specific indication.

After addressing these issues, thorough evaluation of the fetal heart rate tracing includes assessment of the five essential fetal heart rate components: baseline rate, baseline variability, accelerations, presence or absence of decelerations, and changes or trends in the tracing over time.

If necessary, fetal stimulation should be used to provoke accelerations and/or improve fetal heart rate variability, in order to exclude the presence of fetal metabolic acidemia. It is critical to note that fetal stimulation procedures should be performed at times when the fetal heart rate is at baseline. *Neither fetal scalp stimulation nor vibroacoustic stimulation is appropriate during fetal heart rate decelerations or bradycardia.*

EVALUATION OF FIVE ESSENTIAL FETAL HEART RATE COMPONENTS

If all five fetal heart rate components are normal (Box 6-1), there is a very low probability of disrupted fetal oxygenation or evolving metabolic acidemia. As long as there are no other reasons to review the fetal heart rate tracing more frequently (such as fetal growth restriction or preeclampsia), routine intrapartum surveillance is appropriate.

In *low-risk patients*, ACOG/AAP *Guidelines for Prenatal Care* and ACOG *Practice Bulletin* no. 70 recommend that the fetal heart rate tracing be reviewed at least every 30 minutes during the first stage of labor and every 15 minutes during the second stage. *Patients with significant risk factors* should have fetal heart rate

> **BOX 6-1   Five Essential Components of a Fetal Heart Rate Tracing**
>
> 1. Baseline rate
> 2. Baseline variability
> 3. Accelerations
> 4. Decelerations
> 5. Changes or trends over time

tracing evaluation more frequently, every 15 minutes in the first stage and every 5 minutes in the second stage.[4,7]

If one or more of the five fetal heart rate components is abnormal, further evaluation is necessary. Corrective measures may be needed before making a decision regarding management. A practical approach can be summarized as the "A-B-C-Ds" of intrapartum fetal monitoring.

A – Assess the oxygen pathway
B – Begin corrective measures
C – Clear obstacles to rapid delivery
D – Decision to delivery time

A – ASSESS THE OXYGEN PATHWAY

Rapid, systematic assessment of the oxygen pathway from the environment to the fetus can identify possible sources of disrupted oxygenation. As illustrated in Figure 6-1, this pathway includes the maternal lungs, heart, vasculature, uterus, placenta, and umbilical cord. Specific assessment at each point along the oxygen pathway is summarized in Table 6-1. While assessing the oxygen pathway, it is important to consider other conditions that can influence the appearance of a fetal heart rate tracing via mechanisms unrelated to fetal oxygenation (see Table 5-1). If a fetal heart rate abnormality is thought to be related to any of these factors, individualized management is directed at the underlying process. Specific management of each of these conditions is beyond the scope of this book.

B – BEGIN CORRECTIVE MEASURES

At each point along the pathway, appropriate corrective measures should be initiated to optimize oxygen delivery. Specific measures are summarized in Table 6-1. The choice of appropriate corrective measures is based on interpretation of the fetal heart rate tracing as a whole, not on interpretation of individual components out of context. However, it can be refined by acknowledging some specific associations. For example, if variable decelerations are observed, initial attention is focused on the possibility of umbilical cord compression or prolapse. On the other hand, late decelerations usually reflect disruption of the oxygen pathway at a point other than the umbilical cord, and initial attention is focused on maternal cardiac output, blood pressure, and uterine activity.

Specific measures to improve fetal oxygenation are reviewed below.

Supplemental Oxygen

Fetal oxygenation is dependent upon the oxygen content of maternal blood perfusing the intervillous space of the placenta, as discussed in Chapter 2. Administration of supplemental oxygen by nasal cannula or face mask can increase the Po_2 of inspired air, increasing both the partial pressure of oxygen dissolved in maternal blood and the amount of oxygen bound to hemoglobin. This can increase the oxygen concentration gradient across the placental blood–blood barrier and lead to increased fetal Po_2 and oxygen content. Several studies have reported resolution of fetal heart rate abnormalities after administration of supplemental oxygen to the mother, providing indirect evidence of improved fetal oxygenation.[2,11,12,36,55] Direct evidence is provided by fetal pulse oximetry studies demonstrating increased fetal hemoglobin saturation following maternal administration of oxygen. Although the optimal method and duration of oxygen administration is not known, available data support the use of a *non-rebreather face mask to administer oxygen at a rate of 10 L/min for approximately 15 to 30 minutes.*[29,41,55,61]

Maternal Position Changes

There are sound physiologic reasons to avoid the supine position during labor. Supine positioning increases the likelihood that pressure on the inferior vena cava will impair venous return, cardiac output, and perfusion of the intervillous space. It also increases the likelihood that pressure on the descending aorta and/or iliac vessels will impede the delivery of oxygenated blood to the intervillous space.

Prospective fetal pulse oximetry data confirm that *lateral positioning* results in higher fetal hemoglobin saturation levels than does

TABLE 6-1   ABCDs of intrapartum fetal heart rate management

	A Assess Oxygen Pathway	B Begin Corrective Measures		C Clear Obstacles to Rapid Delivery	D Decision to Delivery Time
Lungs	Airway and breathing Breathing technique	Supplemental oxygen if needed Treat pulmonary disorders Alter breathing technique	Facility	Confirm operating room availability and readiness Instruments (vacuum, forceps) Equipment (ultrasound, anesthesia)	Individual facility response time
Heart	Cardiac output Heart rate and rhythm	Consider IV fluid bolus Treat arrhythmia if needed	Staff	Notify appropriate team members Obstetrician Surgical assistant Anesthesiologist Pediatrician/neonatologist Nursing staff	Availability Training Experience
Vasculature	Blood pressure Volume status	Maternal position changes Consider IV fluid bolus Correct hypotension	Mother	Informed consent Consider anesthesia options IV access, urinary catheter Lab results, blood products as needed Abdominal prep if needed Move to operating room if necessary	*Surgical considerations* Prior uterine or abdominal surgery *Medical considerations* Obesity, diabetes, hypertension, SLE *Obstetric considerations* Parity, preeclampsia, clinical pelvimetry

	A Assess Oxygen Pathway	B Begin Corrective Measures		C Clear Obstacles to Rapid Delivery	D Decision to Delivery Time
Uterus	Contraction strength Contraction frequency Baseline uterine rupture Exclude uterine tonus Pushing technique	Stop or reduce uterine stimulants Tocolytic if needed Intrauterine pressure catheter Alter pushing technique	Fetus	Confirm fetal heart rate Consider fetal scalp electrode Confirm gestational age Confirm estimated weight Confirm presentation and position	Rising baseline rate Loss of variability, loss of accelerations Change in deceleration Increasing frequency, depth, duration Fetal growth restriction or macrosomia Presentation and position Prematurity, infection, meconium, anomaly
Placenta	Placental abruption Placenta previa Vasa previa	Rapid delivery if indicated	Labor	Consider tocolytic Consider intrauterine pressure catheter	Estimated time until delivery Protracted labor Arrest disorder Maternal expulsive efforts
Cord	Vaginal exam Cord compression Cord prolapse Amniotic fluid volume Rapid descent Pushing technique	Consider amnioinfusion Elevate fetal head if needed Alter pushing technique Rapid delivery if indicated			

IV, intravenous; *SLE*, systemic lupus erythematosus.
Courtesy David A. Miller, MD.

supine positioning.[1,14,55] In the setting of suspected umbilical cord compression, maternal position changes may result in fetal position changes and relief of pressure on the umbilical cord.

Intravenous Fluid Administration

Optimal uterine perfusion depends upon optimal cardiac output and intravascular volume. Normal blood pressure does not necessarily reflect optimal intravascular volume, venous return, preload, or cardiac output.

An *intravascular bolus of isotonic fluid* can improve cardiac output not only by increasing circulating volume but also by increasing venous return, left ventricular end diastolic pressure, ventricular preload, and ultimately, stroke volume in accordance with the Frank-Starling mechanism. In this way, a relatively small increase in intravascular volume can have a disproportionately greater impact on cardiac output and uterine perfusion.

Simpson[55] demonstrated a significant increase in fetal oxygen saturation following an intravascular isotonic fluid bolus approximating 10% to 20% of blood volume (500-1000 ml). In this study, boluses were administered over 20 minutes to normotensive women without evidence of hypovolemia. The maximum effect was achieved with a 1000-ml bolus, and the beneficial impact on fetal oxygen saturation lasted for more than 30 minutes after the bolus. This study demonstrated that an intravenous fluid bolus of 500 to 1000 ml can improve fetal oxygenation even in an apparently euvolemic patient.

Excessive fluid administration can have serious consequences, and caution must be exercised in patients at risk for volume overload, pulmonary edema, or both. The optimal rate of intravenous fluid administration during labor is not known. Potential maternal and fetal complications argue against administering large-volume intravenous boluses of glucose-containing fluids.

Correcting Maternal Blood Pressure

A number of factors predispose laboring women to transient episodes of hypotension. These include inadequate hydration, insensible fluid losses, supine position resulting in caval compression, decreased venous return and reduced cardiac output, and peripheral vasodilation due to sympathetic blockade during regional anesthesia. Maternal hypotension can reduce uterine perfusion and fetal oxygenation.

Hydration and lateral or Trendelenburg positioning usually correct the blood pressure. However, medication may be necessary. Ephedrine is a sympathomimetic amine with weak α- and β-agonist activity. The primary mechanism of action is displacement of norepinephrine from presynaptic storage vesicles, resulting in release of norepinephrine and stimulation of postsynaptic adrenergic receptors. Ephedrine has no known adverse impact on fetal outcome.

Reducing Uterine Activity

As discussed in detail in previous chapters, excessive uterine activity is a common cause of disrupted fetal oxygenation. It is also a common source of medical-legal liability. A number of terms have been used by clinicians to describe excessive uterine activity. Examples include *hyperstimulation, tachysystole, hypertonus,* and *tetanic contraction.* As discussed previously, these terms are defined inconsistently in the literature and used inconsistently by clinicians.

For the purposes of fetal heart rate management, if an abnormal fetal heart rate pattern is thought to be related to excessive uterine activity, options include *discontinuing uterine stimulants, reducing the dose of uterine stimulants,* and/or *administering uterine relaxants.* Management of uterine activity is discussed in detail in Chapter 4.

Alter Second-Stage Pushing Technique

During the second stage of labor, maternal expulsive efforts can be associated with recurrent variable or prolonged decelerations. Suggested corrective approaches *include open-glottis rather than Valsalva-style pushing, fewer pushing efforts per contraction, shorter individual pushing efforts, pushing with every other or every third contraction, and, in patients with regional anesthesia, pushing only with perceived urge.*[10,50,52,54,60,65]

Amnioinfusion

Intrapartum amnioinfusion involves infusion of isotonic fluid through an intrauterine catheter into the amniotic cavity in order to restore the amniotic fluid volume to normal or near-normal levels. The procedure is intended to relieve intermittent umbilical cord compression that results in variable fetal heart rate decelerations and transient fetal hypoxemia and to dilute thick meconium in attempt to prevent meconium aspiration syndrome.

Amnioinfusion performed for the indication of oligohydramnios and umbilical cord compression reduces the occurrence of variable decelerations and lowers the rate of cesarean delivery.[31] It has no known impact on late decelerations. In a recent large study, amnioinfusion performed for the indication of meconium-stained amniotic fluid alone did not significantly reduce the incidence of meconium aspiration syndrome or perinatal death.[27] The procedure appears to be beneficial in reducing the occurrence of variable decelerations in the setting of oligohydramnios; however, routine amnioinfusion for meconium-stained amniotic fluid without variable decelerations is not recommended by ACOG.[5] A procedure for amnioinfusion is described in Appendix A.

Re-evaluate Fetal Heart Rate After Corrective Measures

After corrective measures, the fetal heart rate tracing is re-evaluated. If all five fetal heart rate components are normal, there is a very low likelihood of disrupted fetal oxygenation and metabolic acidemia, and routine intrapartum surveillance can be resumed. However, if one or more components are persistently abnormal after corrective measures, further evaluation is necessary.

The Next Steps

A fetal heart rate tracing that demonstrates accelerations and/or moderate variability without recurrent decelerations predicts a very low likelihood of significant disruption of fetal oxygenation and evolving metabolic acidemia. However, unless all 5 fetal heart rate components are normal, the fetal heart rate tracing should be evaluated at least every 15 minutes in the first stage of labor and at least every 5 minutes in the second stage. If a fetal heart rate tracing demonstrates recurrent decelerations, the possibility of evolving metabolic acidemia must be considered. Likewise, if the fetal heart rate tracing does not demonstrate accelerations or moderate variability after appropriate corrective measures, evolving metabolic acidemia must be included in the differential diagnosis.

C – CLEAR OBSTACLES TO RAPID DELIVERY

If evolving metabolic acidemia is suspected, it is prudent to plan ahead for the possible need for rapid delivery. This step frequently is overlooked; however, it is a very common area of criticism in the event of an untoward outcome. If rapid delivery becomes necessary, every minute counts. Planning ahead for a potential emergency does not commit the patient to immediate delivery. However, it can help remove some common sources of unnecessary delay in the event that an emergency arises. Every clinical setting is unique. Therefore, a simple checklist can help ensure that important considerations are not overlooked. Consider the individual characteristics of the facility, staff, mother, fetus, and labor. Table 6-1 summarizes steps that can be taken to minimize potential sources of delay.

D – DECISION TO DELIVERY TIME

A number of predictable factors can significantly lengthen the response time and should be taken into consideration when planning further management. As summarized in Table 6-1, these factors include individual characteristics of the facility, staff, mother, fetus, and labor. A realistic estimate of the "decision-to-delivery" time is a key element of the decision process.

After assessing the oxygen pathway, initiating corrective measures to optimize oxygen delivery, and clearing obstacles to rapid delivery, a decision must be made. The decision to allow labor to continue or to proceed with delivery reflects a balance between the interests of the mother and fetus, weighing the perceived benefit of successful vaginal delivery against the perceived risk of developing fetal metabolic acidemia and potential injury before vaginal delivery can be achieved. Clinical circumstance can vary widely, but the question is the same in every case: *"Is vaginal delivery likely to occur before the onset of significant metabolic acidemia and potential injury?"* The answer requires a clinical estimation of two factors: (1) time until vaginal delivery, and (2) time until the onset of significant metabolic acidemia. These factors are discussed below.

Time Until Vaginal Delivery

Clinicians should consider cervical dilation, effacement, station, adequacy of uterine activity, and expected rate of progress to estimate the time until vaginal delivery. Rate of progress can vary with parity, fetal size, position, clinical pelvimetry, maternal expulsive efforts, and many other factors. As a result, the precision of the estimate can vary widely. Nevertheless, a disciplined, systematic approach to the decision-making process requires an ongoing clinical estimate of the anticipated time until vaginal delivery.

Time Until Possible Onset of Metabolic Acidemia

With recurrent decelerations and minimal or absent variability, fetal metabolic acidemia can evolve over approximately 60 to 90 minutes (assuming a previously normal fetal heart rate tracing and no acute events).[26,34,40,46] This process can progress more slowly or more rapidly, depending upon many factors, including the specific fetal heart rate pattern. If accelerations and variability are persistently absent, the fetal heart rate tracing alone cannot reliably exclude metabolic acidemia. On the other hand, if accelerations and/or moderate variability are present, the likelihood of metabolic acidemia is very low.

Increasing frequency, depth and/or duration of decelerations, rising baseline fetal heart rate, loss of variability, and absence of accelerations may indicate more rapid progression to metabolic acidemia. The estimated likelihood of an acute event (prolonged deceleration without recovery) should be weighed against a realistic estimate of "decision-to-delivery" time.

After systematic consideration of each of these factors, a decision can be made with confidence that all significant issues have been addressed. If vaginal delivery is considered unlikely before the onset of metabolic acidemia, the decision process should be documented and the patient counseled regarding the option of operative delivery. The maternal risk of operative delivery should be weighed against the fetal risk of metabolic acidemia and injury. On the other hand, if labor is allowed to continue, the decision process should be documented and the fetal heart rate tracing reviewed at least every 15 minutes in the first stage of labor and every 5 minutes in the second stage.[4,7] Periodic documentation should include interpretation of the fetal heart rate tracing and the corresponding management plan.

Responding to Acute Events

If the fetal heart rate tracing deteriorates suddenly, how quickly must delivery be accomplished in order to prevent injury? The scientific answer to this question is not known. The practical answer is that delivery should be accomplished as rapidly as safely possible. Animal studies and retrospective human studies have suggested time frames ranging from 8 to 26 minutes, depending upon the specific insult and the prior status of the fetus. On the other hand, the "30-minute rule" describes a time frame of 30 minutes from the decision to proceed with operative delivery until the time of the incision. In reality, the standard of care has less to do with the specific number of minutes and seconds than with the perceived reasonableness of the care provided. Rather than focusing on a specific time frame that provides a "safe harbor," energy should be directed at a systematic process of anticipating and eliminating potential sources of unnecessary delay. This highlights the importance of the third step in the management decision model: C – Clear obstacles to rapid delivery.

OTHER METHODS OF FETAL MONITORING

One of the major shortcomings of electronic fetal monitoring is a high rate of false-positive results. Even the most abnormal patterns are poorly predictive of neonatal morbidity. This has led to exploration of alternative methods of evaluating fetal status, including fetal scalp pH determination, scalp stimulation or vibroacoustic stimulation, computer analysis of fetal heart rate, fetal pulse oximetry, and ST segment analysis. In assessing the immediate condition of the newborn, umbilical cord acid–base determination is an adjunct to the Apgar score.

Intrapartum Fetal Scalp pH Determination

Intermittent sampling of scalp blood for pH determination was described in the 1960s and studied extensively in the 1970s. However, its use has been limited by many factors, including the requirements for cervical dilation and membrane rupture, technical difficulty of the procedure, the need for serial pH determinations, and uncertainty regarding interpretation and application of results. It is used infrequently in the U.S. but remains a common practice in many countries outside the U.S.

Fetal Scalp Stimulation and Vibroacoustic Stimulation

A number of studies in the 1980s reported that a fetal heart rate acceleration in response to fetal scalp stimulation or vibroacoustic stimulation was highly predictive of normal scalp blood pH.* A literature review and meta-analysis by Skupski and colleagues[56] confirmed the utility of various methods of intrapartum fetal stimulation, including scalp

---

*15,16,24,25,33,48,57,58

puncture, atraumatic stimulation with an Allis clamp, vibroacoustic stimulation, and digital stimulation.

Procedure

Stimulation methods include the following:

1. Scalp stimulation: Digital pressure and stroking of the fetal scalp for 15 seconds during a vaginal examination
2. Vibration and sound stimulation: Placing an artificial larynx on the maternal abdomen over the fetal head continuously for 1 to 5 seconds

It is crucial for clinicians to recognize that fetal scalp stimulation and vibroacoustic stimulation are diagnostic tools used to provoke fetal heart rate accelerations in order to exclude the presence of fetal metabolic acidemia. As noted previously, fetal stimulation procedures should be performed at times when the fetal heart rate is at baseline. *Neither fetal scalp stimulation nor vibroacoustic stimulation is appropriate during fetal heart rate decelerations or bradycardia.*

Computer Analysis of Fetal Heart Rate

Subjective interpretation of fetal heart rate tracings by visual analysis is hampered by inconsistency and imprecision. In an attempt to overcome this limitation, Dawes and others derived a system of numeric analysis of fetal heart rate.[17] Computer analysis of intrapartum fetal heart rate records has been reported to be more precise than visual assessment.[18,47] However, intrapartum computer analysis has not been shown to improve prediction of neonatal outcome. Keith and colleagues reported the results of a multicenter trial of an intelligent computer system using clinical data in addition to fetal heart rate data.[35] In 50 cases analyzed, the system's performance was indistinguishable from that of 17 expert clinicians. The authors reported that the system was highly consistent, recommended no unnecessary intervention, and performed better than all but two of the experts.

Fetal Pulse Oximetry

Intrapartum reflectance fetal pulse oximetry is a modification of transmission pulse oximetry that indirectly measures the oxygen saturation of hemoglobin in fetal blood. An intrauterine sensor placed in contact with fetal skin uses the differential absorption of red and infrared light by oxygenated and deoxygenated fetal hemoglobin to provide continuous estimation of fetal oxygen saturation. A number of studies have examined the utility of intrapartum fetal pulse oximetry.* Although the technology appears to reduce the incidence of cesarean delivery for fetal indications, no consistent impact on overall cesarean rates or newborn outcomes has been demonstrated. The results of a number of randomized trials led the manufacturer to announce that it would no longer distribute the sensors, effectively withdrawing the product from the market.

ST Segment Analysis

Study of the fetal electrocardiogram has produced some promising results. In sheep, fetal heart rate decelerations that accompanied hypoxemia were associated with characteristic changes in the fetal P-R interval. In 2000, Strachan[59] compared standard electronic fetal monitoring with electronic fetal monitoring plus P-R interval analysis in 1038 women. The groups demonstrated statistically similar rates of operative intervention for presumed fetal distress and no differences in newborn outcomes.

The ST segment of the fetal electrocardiogram represents myocardial repolarization. Myocardial hypoxia can lead to elevation of the ST segment and T wave secondary to catecholamine release, β-adrenoceptor activation, glycogenolysis, and tissue metabolic acidosis.[32,51,64] These observations have led to the development of technology to analyze the fetal electrocardiogram plus the ST waveform (STAN®; Neoventa Medical, Göteborg, Sweden).[9,39] One randomized trial in 2434 patients demonstrated a 46% reduction in operative intervention for fetal distress when ST segment analysis was added to standard electronic fetal monitoring.[63] Operative interventions for dystocia and other indications were not increased. Fewer cases of metabolic acidemia and low 5-minute Apgar scores were observed in the group with electronic fetal monitoring plus ST segment analysis; however, these differences did not reach statistical significance.

Another trial using newer technology included 4966 women randomized to electronic fetal monitoring alone versus electronic fetal monitoring plus ST segment analysis.[3] When analyzed according to intention to treat, the incidence of umbilical artery acidemia was 53% lower in the electronic fetal monitoring plus ST segment analysis group. In the electronic fetal monitoring plus ST segment analysis group, the incidence of cesarean section for fetal distress was 8%, compared to 9% in the group monitored with

---

*13,19-23,28,37,38,43,45,53

electronic fetal monitoring alone ($p = 0.047$). After excluding patients with inadequate fetal heart rate recordings and fetal malformations, these differences were slightly more pronounced.

A recent meta-analysis of four studies, including 9829 women, concluded that adjunctive ST segment analysis was associated with significantly fewer cases of severe metabolic acidemia at birth, fewer cases of neonatal encephalopathy, and fewer operative vaginal deliveries.[42] There were no significant differences in cesarean delivery rates, low 5-minute Apgar scores, or neonatal intensive care unit admissions. This meta-analysis suggests that ST segment analysis might prove to be a useful adjunct to standard electronic fetal monitoring. Although initial results are promising, further research is needed to define the role of this technology in clinical practice.

UMBILICAL CORD ACID–BASE DETERMINATION

Umbilical cord blood gas and pH assessment is a useful adjunct to the Apgar score in assessing the immediate condition of the newborn. There are no contraindications to obtaining cord gases.

ACOG[6] suggests obtaining cord gases in the following clinical situations:

- Cesarean delivery for fetal compromise
- Low 5-minute Apgar score
- Severe growth restriction
- Abnormal fetal heart rate tracing
- Maternal thyroid disease
- Intrapartum fever
- Multifetal gestations

Umbilical *arterial* values reflect fetal condition, whereas umbilical *venous* values reflect placental function. Normal findings preclude the presence of acidemia at, or immediately before, delivery.

Approximate normal values for cord blood are summarized in the following chart.[30,44,49,62]

Approximate Normal Values for Cord Blood

Cord Blood	pH	Pco$_2$ (mm Hg)	Po$_2$ (mm Hg)	Base Deficit (mmol/L)
Artery	7.2-7.3	45-55	15-25	<12
Vein	7.3-7.4	35-45	25-35	<12

The base deficit reflects utilization of buffer bases to help stabilize pH, usually in the setting of peripheral tissue hypoxia, anaerobic metabolism, and accumulation of lactic acid. An umbilical artery pH less than 7.20 usually is considered to define acidemia. Note that a much lower pH (7.0) is defined as the threshold of potential injury.

Acidemia is categorized as respiratory, metabolic, or mixed. Isolated respiratory acidemia is diagnosed when the umbilical artery pH is less than 7.20, the P_{CO_2} is elevated, and the base deficit is <12 mmol/L. This reflects disrupted exchange of blood gases, usually as a transient phenomenon related to umbilical cord compression. Isolated respiratory acidemia is not associated with fetal neurologic injury. Isolated metabolic acidemia is diagnosed when the pH is less than 7.20, the P_{CO_2} is normal, and the base deficit is at least 12 mmol/L. Metabolic acidemia can result from recurrent or prolonged disruption of fetal oxygenation that has progressed to the stage of peripheral tissue hypoxia, anaerobic metabolism, and lactic acid production in excess of buffering capacity. Although most cases of fetal metabolic acidemia do not result in injury, the risk is increased in the setting of significant metabolic acidemia (umbilical artery pH <7.0 and pH ≥ 12 mmol/L). Mixed (respiratory and metabolic) acidemia is diagnosed when the pH is below 7.20, the P_{CO_2} is elevated, and the base deficit is 12 mmol/L or greater. The clinical significance of mixed acidemia is similar to that of isolated metabolic acidemia.

The types of acidemia (respiratory, metabolic, or mixed) are summarized in the following chart.

Types of Acidemia

Blood Gases	Respiratory	Metabolic	Mixed
pH	<7.20	<7.20	<7.20
P_{CO_2}	Elevated	Normal	Elevated
Base deficit	<12 mmol/L	≥ 12 mmol/L	≥ 12 mmol/L

The *procedure* for obtaining umbilical cord blood consists of double-clamping a 10- to 20-cm segment of the umbilical cord immediately after delivery. A specimen should be drawn with a 1-ml plastic syringe that has been flushed with heparin solution (1000 U/ml).

Using separate syringes, draw blood from an umbilical artery first, then from the umbilical vein.

SUMMARY

The *goal* of intrapartum fetal heart rate monitoring is to prevent fetal injury that might result from disruption of normal fetal oxygenation during labor. With respect to fetal oxygenation, there are three *central concepts in the interpretation of intrapartum fetal heart rate tracings.* These concepts are illustrated in Figure 6-1 at the beginning of this chapter.

1. All clinically significant FHR decelerations reflect disruption of oxygen transfer from the environment to the fetus at one or more points along the oxygen pathway.
2. Fetal neurologic injury due to disrupted oxygen transfer does not occur unless it progresses at least to the stage of significant metabolic acidemia (umbilical artery pH <7.0 and base deficit ≥ 12 mmol/L)
3. Significant metabolic acidemia is highly unlikely in the presence of moderate FHR variability and/or accelerations.

A systematic approach to the decision-making process underlying the management of intrapartum fetal heart rate tracings employs these three concepts to decide among *three management options*:

1. Routine intrapartum surveillance
2. Heightened intrapartum surveillance
3. Operative intervention

The decision process uses clinical judgment to *weigh the benefit of vaginal delivery against the risk of fetal metabolic acidemia* and takes into account the individual characteristics of the facility, staff, mother, fetus, and labor. To determine whether vaginal delivery is likely before the onset of significant metabolic acidemia, clinical judgment is used to estimate the following:

- Time until vaginal delivery
- Time until possible onset of metabolic acidemia

After considering these factors, an informed decision can be made with confidence that all key factors have been addressed. This systematic approach does not dictate decisions regarding management. It simply presents a standardized management decision model (Figure 6-2) for the process that helps ensure effective communication, thorough documentation, and ultimately, patient safety.

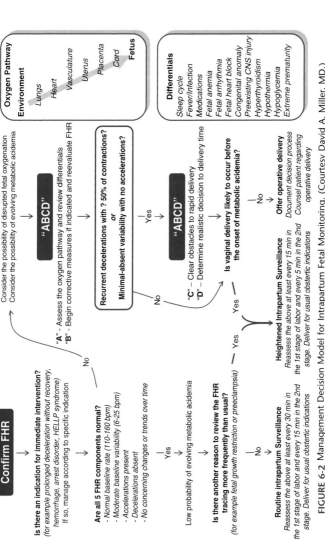

FIGURE 6-2 Management Decision Model for Intrapartum Fetal Monitoring. (Courtesy David A. Miller, MD.)

References

1. Abitbol MM: Supine position in labor and associated fetal heart rate changes, *Am J Obstet Gynecol* 65:481-486, 1985.
2. Althabe O, Schwarcz RL, Pose SV, Escarcena L, Caldeyro-Barcia R: Effects on fetal heart rate and fetal Po_2 of oxygen administration to the mother, *Am J Obstet Gynecol* 98(6):858-870, 1967.
3. Amer-Wåhlin I, Hellsten C, Norén H, Hagberg H, Herbst A, Kjellmer I, Lilja H, Lindoff C, Månsson M, Mårtensson L, Olofsson P, Sundström A, Marsál K: Cardiotocography only versus cardiotocography plus ST analysis of fetal electrocardiogram for intrapartum fetal monitoring: A Swedish randomised controlled trial, *Lancet* 358(9281):534-538, 2001.
4. American Academy of Pediatrics, American College of Obstetricians and Gynecologists: *Guidelines for perinatal care*, ed 6, Washington, DC, 2007, AAP, ACOG.
5. American College of Obstetricians and Gynecologists: Amnioinfusion does not prevent meconium aspiration syndrome, ACOG *Committee Opinion* no. 346, Washington DC, 2006, ACOG.
6. American College of Obstetricians and Gynecologists: Umbilical cord blood gas and acid–base analysis, ACOG *Committee Opinion, Obstet Gynecol* 108(5):1319-1322, 2006.
7. American College of Obstetricians and Gynecologists: Intrapartum fetal heart rate monitoring, ACOG *Practice Bulletin* no.70, *Obstet Gynecol* 106(6):1453-1461, 2005.
8. American College of Obstetricians and Gynecologists Task Force on Neonatal Encephalopathy and Cerebral Palsy, American College of Obstetricians and Gynecologists, American Academy of Pediatrics: *Neonatal encephalopathy and cerebral palsy: Defining the pathogenesis and pathophysiology*, Washington, DC, 2003, ACOG, AAP.
9. Arulkumaran S, Lilja H, Lindecrantz K, Ratnam SS, Thavarasah AS, Rosén KG: Fetal ECG waveform analysis should improve fetal surveillance in labour, *J Perinatal Med* 18(1):13-22, 1990.
10. Association of Women's Health, Obstetric and Neonatal Nurses: *Nursing management of the second stage of labor. Evidence-based clinical practice guideline*, Washington, DC, 2000, AWHONN.
11. Bartnicki J, Saling E: Influence of maternal oxygen administration on the computer-analysed fetal heart rate patterns in small-for-gestational-age fetuses, *Gynecol Obstet Invest* 37(3):172-175, 1994.
12. Bartnicki J, Saling E: The influence of maternal oxygen administration on the fetus, *Int J Gynaecol Obstet* 45(2):87-95, 1994.
13. Bloom SL, Spong CY, Thom E, Varner MW, Rouse DJ, Weininger S, Ramin SM, Caritis SN, Peaceman A, Sorokin Y, Sciscione A, Carpenter M, Mercer B, Thorp J, Malone F, Harper M, Iams J, Anderson G; National Institute of Child Health and Human Development Maternal-Fetal Medicine Units Network: Fetal pulse oximetry and cesarean delivery, *N Engl J Med* 355(21):2195, 2202, 2006.

14. Carbonne B, Benachi A, Leveque ML, Cabrol D, Papiernik E: Maternal position during labor: Effects on fetal oxygen saturation measured by pulse oximetry, *Obstet Gynecol* 88(5):797-800, 1996.
15. Clark SL, Gimovsky ML, Miller FC: Fetal heart rate response to scalp blood sampling, *Am J Obstet Gynecol* 144(6):706-708, 1982.
16. Clark SL, Gimovsky ML, Miller FC: The scalp stimulation test: A clinical alternative to fetal scalp blood sampling, *Am J Obstet Gynecol* 148 (3):274-277, 1984.
17. Dawes GS: Computerised analysis of the fetal heart rate, *Eur J Obstet Gynecol Reprod Biol* 42(Suppl):S5-S8, 1991.
18. Dawes GS, Moulden M, Sheil O, Redman CWG: Approximate entropy, a statistic of regularity, applied to fetal heart rate data before and during labor, *Obstet Gynecol* 80(5):763-768, 1992.
19. Dildy GA, Clark SL, Loucks CA: Intrapartum fetal pulse oximetry: Past, present, and future, *Am J Obstet Gynecol* 175(1):1-9, 1996.
20. Dildy GA, Clark SL, Loucks CA: Preliminary experience with intrapartum fetal pulse oximetry in humans, *Obstet Gynecol* 81(4):630-635, 1993.
21. Dildy GA, van den Berg PP, Katz M, Clark SL, Jongsma HW, Nijhuis JG, Loucks CA: Intrapartum fetal pulse oximetry: fetal oxygen saturation trends during labor and relation to delivery outcome, *Am J Obstet Gynecol* 171(3):679-684, 1994.
22. Dildy GA, Thorp JA, Yeast JD, Clark SL: The relationship between oxygen saturation and pH in umbilical blood: Implications for intrapartum fetal oxygen saturation monitoring, *Am J Obstet Gynecol* 175(3 Pt 1): 682-687, 1996.
23. East CE, Brennecke SP, King JF, Chan FY, Colditz PB: The effect of intrapartum fetal pulse oximetry, in the presence of a nonreassuring fetal heart rate pattern, on operative delivery rates: A multicenter, randomized, controlled trial (the FOREMOST trial), *Am J Obstet Gynecol* 194 (3):606.e1-606.e16, 2006.
24. Edersheim TG, Hutson JM, Druzin ML, Kogut EA: Fetal heart rate response to vibratory acoustic stimulation predicts fetal pH in labor, *Am J Obstet Gynecol* 157(6):1557-1560, 1987.
25. Elimian A, Figueroa R, Tejani N: Intrapartum assessment of fetal well-being: a comparison of scalp stimulation with scalp blood pH sampling, *Obstet Gynecol* 89(3):373-376.
26. Fleischer A, Schulman H, Jagani N, Mitchell J, Randolph G: The development of fetal acidosis in the presence of an abnormal fetal heart rate tracing. I. The average for gestational age fetus, *Am J Obstet Gynecol* 144(1):55-60, 1982.
27. Fraser WD, Hofmeyr J, Lede R, Faron G, Alexander S, Goffinet F, Ohlsson A, Goulet C, Turcot-Lemay L, Prendiville W, Marcoux S, Laperrière L, Roy C, Petrou S, Xu HR, Wei B; Amnioinfusion Trial Group: Amnioinfusion for the prevention of the meconium aspiration syndrome, *N Engl J Med* 353(9):909-917, 2005.

28. Garite TJ, Dildy GA, McNamara H, Nageotte MP, Boehm FH, Dellinger EH, Knuppel RA, Porreco RP, Miller HS, Sunderji S, Varner MW, Swedlow DB: A multicenter controlled trial of fetal pulse oximetry in the intrapartum management of nonreassuring fetal heart rate patterns, *Am J Obstet Gynecol* 183(5):1049-1058, 2000.

29. Haydon ML, Gorenberg DM, Nageotte MP, Ghamsary M, Rumney PJ, Patillo C, Garite TJ: The effect of maternal oxygen administration on fetal pulse oximetry during labor in fetuses with nonreassuring fetal heart rate patterns, *Am J Obstet Gynecol* 195(3):735-738, 2006.

30. Helwig JT, Parer JT, Kilpatrick SJ, Laros RK: Umbilical cord blood acid–base state: What is normal? *Am J Obstet Gynecol* 174(6):1807-1812, 1996.

31. Hofmeyr GJ: Amnioinfusion for potential or suspected umbilical cord compression in labour, *Cochrane Database Syst Rev* 2:CD000013, 2000.

32. Hökegård KH, Eriksson BO, Kjellemer I, Magno R, Rosén KG: Myocardial metabolism in relation to electrocardiographic changes and cardiac function during graded hypoxia in the fetal lamb, *Acta Physiol Scand* 113(1):1-7, 1981.

33. Ingemarsson I, Arulkumaran S: Reactive fetal heart rate response to VAS in fetuses with low scalp blood pH, *Br J Obstet Gynaecol* 96(5):562-565, 1989.

34. Ingemarsson I, Herbst A, Thorgren-Jerneck K: Long-term outcome after umbilical artery acidemia at term birth: Influence of gender and fetal heart rate abnormalities, *Br J Obstet Gynaecol* 104(10):1123-1127, 1997.

35. Keith RDF, Beckly S, Garibaldi JM, Westgate JA, Ifeachor EC, Greene KR: A multicentre comparative study of 17 experts and an intelligent computer system for managing labour using the cardiotocogram, *Br J Obstet Gynaecol* 102(9):688-700, 1995.

36. Khazin AF, Hon EH, Hehre FW: Effects of maternal hyperoxia on the fetus I. Oxygen tension, *Am J Obstet Gynecol* 109(4):628-637, 1971.

37. Klauser CK, Christensen EE, Chauhan SP, Bufkin L, Magann EF, Bofill JA, Morrison JC: Use of fetal pulse oximetry among high-risk women in labor: A randomized clinical trial, *Am J Obstet Gynecol* 192(16):1810-1819, 2005.

38. Kuhnert M, Seelbach-Goebel G, Butterwegge M: Predictive agreement between the fetal arterial oxygen saturation and fetal scalp pH: Results of the German multicenter study, *Am J Obstet Gynecol* 178(2):330-335, 1998.

39. Lilja H, Karlsson K, Lindecrantz K, Rosén KG: Microprocessor based waveform analysis of the fetal electrocardiogram during labor, *Int J Gynecol Obstet* 30:109-116, 1989.

40. Low JA, Galbraith RS, Muir DW, Killen HL, Pater EA, Karchmar EJ: Factors associated with motor and cognitive deficits in children after intrapartum fetal hypoxia, *Am J Obstet Gynecol* 148:533-539, 1982.

41. McNamara H, Johnson N, Lilford R: The effect on fetal arteriolar oxygen saturation resulting from giving oxygen to the mother measured by pulse oximetry, *Br J Obstet Gynaecol* 100(5):446-449, 1993.

42. Neilson JP: Fetal electrocardiogram (ECG) for fetal monitoring during labour, *Cochrane Database Syst Rev* 3:CD000116, 2006.

43. Nijland R, Jongsma HW, Nijhuis JG, van den Berg PP, Oeseburg B: Arterial oxygen saturation in relation to metabolic acidosis in fetal lambs, *Am J Obstet Gynecol* 172(3):810-819, 1995.

44. Nodwell A, Carmichael L, Ross M, Richardson B: Placental compared with umbilical cord blood to assess fetal blood gas and acid-base status, *Obstet Gynecol* 105(1):129-138, 2005.

45. Oeseburg B, Ringnalda BEM, Crevels J, Jongsma HW, Mannheimer P, Menssen J, Nijhuis JG: Fetal oxygenation in chronic maternal hypoxia: What's critical? *Adv Exp Med Biol* 317:499-502, 1992.

46. Parer JT, King T, Flanders S, Fox M, Kilpatrick SJ: Fetal acidemia and electronic fetal heart rate patterns. Is there evidence of an association? *J Matern Fetal Neonatal Med* 19(2):289-294, 2006.

47. Pello LC, Rosevear BM, Dawes GS, Moulden M, Redman CW: Compu-terized fetal heart rate analysis in labor, *Obstet Gynecol* 78(4):602-610, 1991.

48. Polzin GB, Blakemore KJ, Petrie RH, Amon E: Fetal vibro-acoustic stimulation: Magnitude and duration of fetal heart rate accelerations as a marker of fetal health, *Obstet Gynecol* 72(4):621-626, 1988.

49. Richardson, B, Nodwell A; Webster K, Alshimmiri M, Gagnon R, Natale R: Fetal oxygen saturation and fractional extraction at birth and the relationship to measures of acidosis, *Am J Obstet Gynecol* 178 (3):572-579, 1998.

50. Roberts J, Hanson J: Best practices in second stage labor care: Maternal bearing down and positioning, *J Midwifery Women's Health* 52(3):238-245, 2007.

51. Rosén KG, Dagbjartsson A, Henriksson BA, Lagercrantz H, Kjellmer I: The relationship between circulating catecholamine and ST waveform in the fetal lamb electrocardiogram during hypoxia, *Am J Obstet Gynecol* 149(2):190-195, 1984.

52. Sameshima H, Ikenoue T: Predictive value of late decelerations for fetal acidemia in unselective low-risk pregnancies, *Am J Perinatol* 22(1): 19-23, 2005.

53. Seelbach-Gobel B, Butterwegge M, Kuhnert M, Heupel M: Fetal reflec-tance pulse oximetry sub partu. Experiences – prognostic significance and consequences – goals, *Zeitschr Geburtshilfe Perinatol* 198:67-71, 1994.

54. Simpson KR, James DC: Effects of immediate versus delayed pushing during second-stage labor on fetal well-being: A randomized clinical trial, *Nurs Res* 54(3):149-157, 2005.

55. Simpson KR, James DC: Efficacy of intrauterine resuscitation techni-ques in improving fetal oxygen status during labor, *Obstet Gynecol* 105(6):1362-1368, 2005.

56. Skupski DW, Rosenberg CR, Eglington GS: Intrapartum fetal stimula-tion tests: A meta-analysis, *Obstet Gynecol* 99(1):129-134, 2002.

57. Smith CV, Nguyen HN, Phelan JP, Paul RH: Intrapartum assessment of fetal well-being: A comparison of fetal acoustic stimulation with acid-base determinations, *Am J Obstet Gynecol* 155(4):726-728, 1986.

58. Spencer JA: Predictive value of a fetal heart rate acceleration at the time of fetal blood sampling in labour, *J Perinat Med* 19(3):207-215, 1991.

59. Strachan BK, van Wijngaarden WJ, Sahota D, Chang A, James DK: Cardiotocography only versus cardiotocography plus PR-interval analysis in intrapartum surveillance: A randomized, multicentre trial, *Lancet* 355 (9202):456-459, 2000.

60. Terek MC, Gundem G, Kazandi M, Sendag F, Akercan F: Different types of variable decelerations and their effects to neonatal outcome, *Singapore Med J* 44(5):243-247, 2003.

61. Thorp JA, Trobough T, Evans R, Hedrick J, Yeast JD: The effect of maternal oxygen administration during the second stage of labor on umbilical cord blood gas values: A randomized controlled prospective trial, *Am J Obstet Gynecol* 172:46-74, 1995.

62. Victory R, Penava D, Da Silva O, Natale R, Richardson B: Umbilical cord pH and base excess values in relation to adverse outcome events for infants delivering at term, *Am J Obstet Gynecol* 191(6):2021-2028, 2004.

63. Westgate J, Harris M, Curnow JS, Greene KR: Plymouth randomized trial of cardiotocogram only versus ST waveform plus cardiotogram for intrapartum monitoring in 2400 cases, *Am J Obstet Gynecol* 169 (5):1151-1160, 1993.

64. Widmark C, Jansson T, Lindecrantz K, Rosén KG: ECG waveform, short term heart rate variability and plasma catecholamine concentrations in response to hypoxia in intrauterine growth retarded guinea pig fetuses, *J Dev Physiol* 15(3):161-168, 1991.

65. Williams KP, Galerneau F: Intrapartum fetal heart rate patterns in the prediction of neonatal acidemia, *Am J Obstet Gynecol* 188(3):820-823, 2003.

Influence of Gestational Age on Fetal Heart Rate

P hysiologic characteristics of the preterm fetus may differ from those of the term fetus. Gestational age influences the baseline heart rate, the appearance and amplitude of accelerations, and may influence variability. Monitoring of the smaller fetus and uterus can present significant challenges in both collection and interpretation of data. Furthermore, the postterm fetus has gestational-age–related characteristics that differ from those of the preterm and term fetus. This chapter reviews available data regarding the physiologic characteristics of the preterm and postterm fetus with emphasis on interpretation of fetal monitoring data and assessment of fetal status.

THE PRETERM FETUS

The incidence of preterm birth in the United States has risen 20% since 1990 and reached a new high of 12.7%, according to 2005 natality data.[11] The most marked increase was in late preterm births (34-36 weeks), which rose from 7.3% in 1990 to 9.1% in 2005 (Figure 7-1). Data indicate that nonreassuring fetal heart rate (FHR) patterns in the preterm fetus may have greater predictive value related to survival.[4,5,22] These findings underscore the importance of clinical acumen regarding the heart rate patterns of preterm fetuses, which differ in some ways from those of full-term fetuses.

The following fetal heart rate characteristics have been described in the preterm fetus; however, quantitative data are limited.

- Average baseline rate is slightly higher.
- Minimal variability may be observed in extremely premature fetuses.
- Accelerations may be of lower amplitude (10 beats per minute × 10 sec) until 32 weeks.
- Accelerations may be less frequent in extremely premature fetuses.

- Episodic decelerations may occur unrelated to hypoxia in preterm fetuses.
- Periodic decelerations may be more frequent during labor.

Baseline Fetal Heart Rate in the Preterm Fetus

The baseline fetal heart rate decreases as gestational age increases. In a preterm fetus, a baseline rate close to 160 beats per minute can be normal but must be interpreted with caution. Tachycardia (fetal heart rate baseline >160) should always be evaluated using a systematic approach (see Chapter 6) regardless of gestational age.

Periodic and Episodic Heart Rate Changes in the Preterm Fetus

Accelerations of the fetal heart rate in association with fetal movement begin in the second trimester of pregnancy. Before approximately 30 weeks of gestation, spontaneous decelerations may occur in association with fetal activity.[28]

Maturation of the physiologic mechanisms responsible for fetal heart rate accelerations is related to advancing gestational age. As a result, a nonstress test performed before 32 weeks of gestation may be "non-reactive" by criteria used for term gestations without

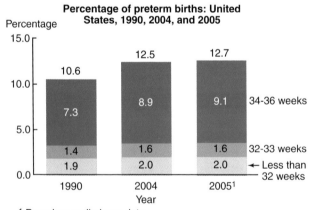

¹ Based on preliminary data.
SOURCE: CDC/NCHS, National Vital Statistics System

FIGURE 7-1 Increase in preterm births in the United States 1990–2005.

signaling disrupted fetal oxygenation or metabolic acidemia.[1] Premature fetuses may not demonstrate accelerations of 15 beats per minute lasting 15 seconds; therefore, before 32 weeks of gestation, a fetal heart rate acceleration is defined by a peak of 10 beats per minute or more above the baseline and a duration of 10 seconds or more from onset to offset.[3,26]

If additional information is needed regarding fetal status, ultrasound visualization of normal fetal breathing, movement, tone, and amniotic fluid volume is highly predictive of the absence of metabolic acidemia.[13,17,19-21] Fetal breathing movements have been reported to increase with increasing maternal P_{CO_2} and decrease with low P_{CO_2}.[17]

As summarized below, a number of fetal heart rate changes may occur as the fetus approaches term; these are related to advancing gestational age and fetal maturation.

- Decrease in baseline rate toward the lower end of normal range
- Increase in variability
- Increase in number, frequency, and amplitude of accelerations
- Possible decrease in the number of spontaneous decelerations

Behavior States in the Preterm Fetus

Four fetal behavioral states have been described and verified by real-time ultrasound (Table 7-1). The fetus may cycle between these states, as demonstrated in Figure 7-2.

Near term, the fetus can remain in one state for approximately 20 to 40 minutes.[14] Clinically, intermittent fetal sleep cycles may result in periods of decreased variability and infrequent accelerations. Pathologic causes must be excluded before these fetal heart rate observations can safely be attributed to benign changes in behavioral state. Alternatively, frequent accelerations during the active 4F state can confound reliable assignment of baseline rate. In that event, simultaneous evaluation of the fetal heart rate tracing and fetal movement can help differentiate baseline rate (between fetal movements) from accelerations (during fetal movements).

Preterm Uterine Activity

Preterm uterine activity monitoring may be technically challenging. The smaller uterus may not accommodate effective placement of both toco and ultrasound transducers. Low-amplitude, high-frequency

TABLE 7-1   Fetal Behavioral States

State	Behavior	Associated FHR Pattern
1F: Quiet sleep	Absence of rapid eye movement (REM); infrequent body and startle movements; rhythmic mouthing movements	Regular/stable fetal heart rate; minimal variability; rare accelerations with fetal movement (FM)
2F: Active sleep	Frequent body movements; abrupt head and limb movement; REM	Minimal to moderate variability; frequent accelerations with FM
3F: Quiet awake	Infrequent body movements, REM	Moderate variability
4F: Active awake	Continuous and vigorous movement	Moderate to marked variability; frequent accelerations fusing into tachycardia

From Blackburn ST: *Maternal, fetal, and neonatal physiology: A clinical perspective,* ed 3, St Louis, 2007, Saunders; Druzin ML, Gabbe SG, Reed KL: Antepartum fetal evaluation. In Gabbe SG, Niebyl JR, Simpson JL, editors: *Obstetrics: Normal and problem pregnancies,* ed 5, New York, 2007, Churchill Livingstone; Harman CR, Menticoglou S, Manning FA: Assessing fetal health. In James KD, Steer J, Weiner CP, Gonic B, editors: *High risk pregnancy: Management options,* ed 3, Philadelphia, 2005, Bailliere Tindall; Richardson BS, Gagnon R: Fetal breathing and body movements. In Creasy RK, Resnik R, Iams JD, editors: *Maternal-fetal medicine: Principals and practice,* ed 5, Philadelphia, 2004, Saunders.

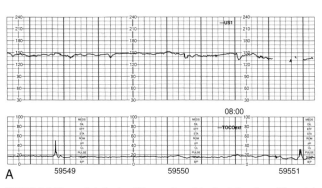

FIGURE 7-2 The cyclic behavior of the near-term fetus (gestational age, 35 weeks). A significant difference in both variability and the presence of accelerations correlates with sleep and wake sates. **A.** 1F behavior is demonstrated with the quiet sleep state. Accelerations are absent and the variability is decreased.

Continued

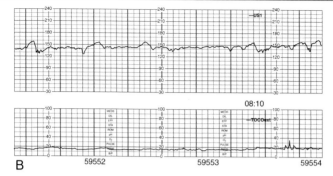

FIGURE 7-2 cont'd **B.** As the fetus has frequent body movements during active sleep (2F), accelerations are evidenced and the variability increases to become moderate.

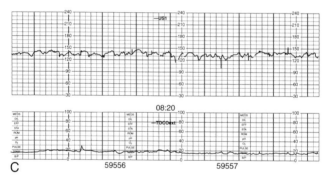

C. In the quiet awake state (3F), moderate variability continues with only occasional accelerations.

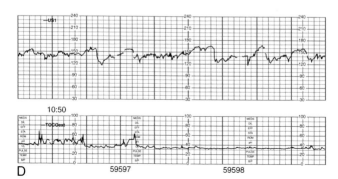

D. In the 4F state, the fetus is vigorous and awake, variability increases, and accelerations merge and coalesce.

uterine contractions, frequently called "uterine irritability," are not uncommon before term. In most cases, these contractions are clinically benign; however, occasionally they may progress to preterm labor contractions or may signal evolving placental abruption. Contractions that do not resolve must be evaluated in the context of the clinical presentation and fetal heart rate observations. Painful uterine contractions in a pregnancy at low risk for preterm delivery can make accurate diagnosis difficult. Because preterm delivery is associated with significant morbidity and mortality, health care providers often exercise caution and administer tocolytic medications in this situation.

Tocolytic Agents and Effect on Fetal Heart Rate

Indomethacin

Most tocolytic protocols are designed to minimize maternal side effects. In contrast, the protocols for administering indomethacin (Indocin), a prostaglandin synthetase inhibitor, are designed to minimize fetal risks of constriction of the ductus arteriosus and decreased renal function resulting in a decrease in amniotic fluid volume. Therapy is often limited to 48 hours and to gestational ages below 30 to 32 weeks. Assessment of amniotic fluid volume is performed at the initiation of therapy and whenever a decision is made to prolong therapy. Prolonged indomethacin therapy is often accompanied by daily sonographic assessment of the possibility of developing oligohydramnios and constriction of the fetal ductus arteriosus. If oligohydramnios develops, the fetal heart rate tracing may reveal variable decelerations, reflecting transient umbilical cord compression.

Nifedipine

The calcium-channel blocker nifedipine (Procardia) may cause a mild increase in maternal heart rate and a modest decrease in diastolic blood pressure. Any medication that reduces maternal blood pressure has the potential to interfere with normal maternal perfusion of the intervillous space. As discussed in Chapter 5, recurrent or sustained disruption of fetal oxygenation can result in fetal heart rate changes ranging from decelerations to loss of variability, loss of accelerations, and a rising baseline rate.

Terbutaline

The beta-sympathomimetic terbutaline (Brethine) causes maternal tachycardia and an increase in oxygen consumption. Fetal tachycardia often parallels maternal tachycardia and may be associated with decreased variability. With prolonged use, fetal arrhythmia may develop as well.

Magnesium Sulfate

Magnesium sulfate, the most commonly used tocolytic in the United States, has been associated with decreased baseline variability and accelerations. Pathologic causes should be excluded before these changes are attributed to magnesium sulfate therapy. Fetal tactile or vibroacoustic stimulation can provoke accelerations and may improve variability.[10,12,30,32] Ultrasound assessment of fetal breathing, movement, tone, and amniotic fluid volume (biophysical profile) may provide useful information regarding the likelihood of fetal metabolic acidemia.[13,19-21]

Other Medications

Decreased fetal heart rate variability has been described in association with betamethasone administration, but not with dexamethasone.[3]

Monitoring the Preterm Fetus

Antepartum Testing

Some maternal conditions, for example, poorly controlled hypertension or systemic lupus erythematosus, may require early initiation of antepartum testing. However, in general, antepartum testing is not initiated before 24 to 26 weeks. For most medical indications, testing is initiated by 32 to 34 weeks. Fetal death resulting from disrupted oxygenation is uncommon prior to 32 to 34 weeks. In view of the relatively high false-positive rates of most testing protocols, earlier initiation of testing should be expected to increase the incidence of unnecessary intervention and iatrogenic prematurity, with their attendant complications.

Antepartum Monitoring

Continuous monitoring is frequently performed during tocolytic therapy for presumed preterm labor or during expectant management of conditions such as preterm premature membrane rupture or preeclampsia. Any time fetal heart rate monitoring is performed prior to term, there is a risk that a false-positive "abnormal" fetal heart rate tracing will prompt unnecessary delivery of an uncompromised fetus. The earlier in gestation this occurs, the higher the likelihood of serious iatrogenic sequelae of prematurity. This risk must be balanced against the anticipated benefits of the information obtained from the monitor. Fetal monitoring may offer the benefit of early detection of disrupted fetal oxygenation so that operative intervention can be performed in a timely fashion. However, in the case of extreme prematurity, the management plan might not include the option of operative intervention. Nevertheless, there are a number of conservative measures short of operative intervention that might benefit the fetus, including maternal oxygen administration, correcting hypotension, intravenous fluid bolus, position changes, discontinuing or reducing the dose of uterine stimulants, administering uterine relaxants, or performing amnioinfusion. Prior to term, the decision to initiate or discontinue fetal monitoring or to perform continuous versus intermittent monitoring is made on an individual basis after a realistic assessment of the anticipated risks, benefits, limitations, and alternatives. It is always appropriate to include the patient in the decision-making process.

Intrapartum Monitoring

Except in cases of intractable preterm labor prior to viability, intrapartum management includes continuous monitoring with regular review of the fetal heart rate tracing as outlined in Chapter 6. In a preterm fetus, disrupted oxygenation may progress more rapidly to metabolic acidemia and potential injury. In addition, the possibility of infection must be entertained in all cases of preterm labor and/or premature membrane rupture. The effects of infection and/or inflammation on the fetal heart rate tracing are incompletely understood. In a premature fetus, the fetal heart rate tracing may be less reliable in predicting metabolic acidemia and outcome. All of these factors must be taken into consideration when interpreting the fetal heart rate tracing and planning intrapartum management of the preterm fetus.

THE POSTTERM FETUS

Postterm pregnancy is defined as a gestation of more than 42 weeks, or 294 days from the last menstrual period. The incidence of postterm pregnancy is approximately 10%. Although the precise magnitude of risk is not known, fetal and neonatal morbidity and mortality increase as pregnancy advances beyond 42 weeks. Antepartum testing in postterm pregnancy is reviewed in Chapter 9. The definition, interpretation, and management of intrapartum fetal heart rate patterns in the postterm fetus do not differ from those in the term fetus.

Risks Associated With Postterm Pregnancy

Macrosomia

Macrosomia is defined as a birthweight greater than 4500 g. Many reports have described an increased incidence of this complication in the postterm population. Birthweights exceeding 4500 g have been reported in 2.8% to 5.4% of postterm infants compared to 0.8% of term infants.[9,29,35] At any gestational age, fetal macrosomia is associated with increased risks of shoulder dystocia, birth trauma, and cesarean delivery.[15,33,34]

Oligohydramnios

Oligohydramnios is observed with increased frequency in the postterm gestation. Sonographic descriptions include the subjective impression of decreased fluid volume, measurement of the deepest vertical fluid pocket, and calculation of the amniotic fluid index. The amniotic fluid index is a semiquantitative assessment of amniotic fluid volume, defined as the sum of the measurements of the deepest, vertical, cord-free pockets in each uterine quadrant. Beyond 40 weeks, the amniotic fluid index can decline by as much as 30% to 50%.[6,27] The increased morbidity associated with oligohydramnios is well documented and includes increased incidences of meconium-stained amniotic fluid and cesarean section for fetal indications. Other associations include low Apgar scores and umbilical artery pH values, increased rates of meconium aspiration syndrome, and umbilical cord compression leading to variable decelerations.

Meconium

Numerous reports have described an increased frequency of meconium passage in postterm pregnancies. The incidence of 25% to 30% represents a two-fold increase over that observed at term. However, meconium passage alone is not a reliable indicator of fetal compromise. In many cases, meconium passage may simply reflect a maturing fetus. Alternatively, it may reflect stimulation of the vagal system by umbilical cord compression or transient hypoxemia. Even when meconium passage is not secondary to these causes, it poses the risk of meconium aspiration syndrome. The risk is compounded by diminished amniotic fluid volume, resulting in thick, undiluted meconium that is more likely to obstruct the airways. The incidence of meconium aspiration syndrome in the presence of meconium-stained amniotic fluid may be as high as 2%.[8]

As discussed in Chapter 6, the American College of Obstetricians and Gynecologists (ACOG)[2] does not recommend routine amnioinfusion for meconium-stained amniotic fluid. However, amnioinfusion remains appropriate for treatment of variable decelerations.

Postmaturity or Dysmaturity

Approximately 10% to 20% of postterm fetuses can exhibit clinical signs of the "postmaturity" or "dysmaturity" syndrome, including reduced subcutaneous tissue; dry, wrinkled, peeling skin; and meconium staining.[7] Additional observations include hypothermia, hypoglycemia, polycythemia, and hyperviscosity. These findings, present in approximately 3% of term infants, are thought to reflect subacute disruption of normal placental transfer of oxygen and nutrients, leading to nutritional deprivation, fetal wasting, decreased fat and glycogen stores, oligohydramnios, and chronic hypoxemia with compensatory hematopoiesis.

Intrapartum Management

Intrapartum management of the postterm pregnancy should include sonographic estimation of fetal weight and amniotic fluid volume. An estimated fetal weight of more than 4500 g should prompt a frank discussion with the patient regarding the risks associated with macrosomia, including shoulder dystocia and associated birth trauma. Elective cesarean delivery may be considered. At estimated weights between 4000 and 4500 g, the decision to attempt a vaginal delivery should take into account such factors as obstetric history, clinical pelvimetry, maternal obesity, and diabetes. In the intrapartum period, the postterm fetus is at increased risk for meconium passage, oligohydramnios, and umbilical cord compression. Continuous fetal heart rate monitoring is recommended.

Oligohydramnios is associated with thick meconium, intrapartum variable decelerations, and cesarean section for fetal indications. In the presence of meconium and variable decelerations, intrapartum saline amnioinfusion may reduce the frequency of decelerations and the incidence of cesarean section for fetal indications.[16,18,23-25,31]

SUMMARY

Maturation of the physiologic mechanisms responsible for regulation of the fetal heart rate is associated with characteristic changes in the fetal heart rate tracing. In addition, many factors associated with pre-term and postterm pregnancy can influence the appearance of the fetal heart rate tracing, including medications, infection, inflammation, and oligohydramnios. All of these factors must be taken into consideration when interpreting the fetal heart rate tracing and planning management of pregnancies before and after term.

References

1. American Academy of Pediatrics, American College of Obstetricians and Gynecologists: *Guidelines for perinatal care*, ed 6, Washington, DC, 2007, AAP, ACOG.

2. American College of Obstetricians and Gynecologists: Amnioinfusion does not prevent meconium aspiration syndrome, ACOG *Committee Opinion* no. 346, Washington, DC, 2006, ACOG.

3. American College of Obstetricians and Gynecologists: Intrapartum fetal heart rate monitoring, ACOG *Practice Bulletin* no.70, *Obstet Gynecol* 106(6):1453-1461, 2005.

4. Ayoubi JM, Audibert F, Boithias C, Zupan V, Taylor S, Bosson JL, Frydman R: Perinatal factors affecting survival and survival without disability of extreme premature infants at two years of age, *Eur J Obstet Gynecol Reprod Biol* 105(2):124-131, 2002.

5. Ayoubi JM, Audibert F, Vial M, Pons JC, Taylor S, Frydman R: Fetal heart rate and survival of the very premature newborn, *Am J Obstet Gynecol* 187(4):1026-1030, 2002.

6. Beischer NA, Brown JB, Townsend L: Studies in prolonged pregnancy. III. Amniocentesis in prolonged pregnancy, *Am J Obstet Gynecol* 103 (4):496-503, 1969.

7. Clifford SH: Postmaturity, with placental dysfunction: Clinical syndromes and pathologic findings, *J Pediatr* 44(1):1-13, 1954.

8. Davis RO, Philips JB, Harris BA, Wilson ER, Huddleston JF: Fatal meconium aspiration syndrome occurring despite airway management considered appropriate, *Am J Obstet Gynecol* 151(6):731-736, 1985.

9. Eden RD, Seifert LS, Winegar A, Spellacy WN: Perinatal characteristics of uncomplicated postdate pregnancies, *Obstet Gynecol* 69(3 Pt 1):296-299, 1987.

10. Edersheim TG, Hutson JM, Druzin ML, Kogut EA: Fetal heart rate response to vibratory acoustic stimulation predicts fetal pH in labor, *Am J Obstet Gynecol* 157(6):1557-1560, 1987.

11. Hamilton BE, Martin JA, Ventura SJ: *Births: Preliminary data for 2005. Health E-Stats.* Released November 21, 2006. Accessed September 7, 2008, from www.cdc.gov/nchs/products/pubs/pubd/hestats/prelimbirths05/prelimbirths05.htm.

12. Ingemarsson I, Arulkumaran S: Reactive fetal heart rate response to VAS in fetuses with low scalp blood pH, *Br J Obstet Gynaecol* 96(5):562-565, 1989.

13. Johnson JM, Harman CR, Lange IR, Manning FA: Biophysical profile scoring in the management of postterm pregnancy: An analysis of 307 patients, *Am J Obstet Gynecol* 154(2):269-273, 1986.

14. Johnson T, Besinger RE, Thomas RL New clues to fetal behavior and well being, *Contemp Ob/Gyn* 31(5):108-123, 1988.

15. Lazer S, Biale Y, Mazor M, Lewenthal H, Insler V: Complications associated with the macrosomic fetus, *J Reprod Med* 31(6):501-505, 1986.

16. Lo KW, Rogers M: A controlled trial of amnioinfusion: the prevention of meconium aspiration in labour, *Aust N Z J Obstet Gynaecol* 33(1):51-54, 1993.

17. Lowe N, Reiss R: Parturition and fetal adaptation, *J Obstet Gynecol Neonatal Nurs* 25(4):339-349, 1996.

18. Macri CJ, Schrimmer DB, Leung A, Greenspoon JS, Paul RH: Prophylactic amnioinfusion improves outcome of pregnancy complicated by thick meconium and oligohydramnios, *Am J Obstet Gynecol* 167 (4 Pt 1):117-121, 1992.

19. Manning FA, Morrison I, Harman CR, Lange IR, Menticoglou S: Fetal assessment based on fetal biophysical profile scoring: experience in 19,221 referred high-risk pregnancies. II. An analysis of false-negative fetal deaths, *Am J Obstet Gynecol* 157(4 Pt 1):880-884, 1987.

20. Manning FA, Morrison I, Lange I, Harman CR, Chamberlain PF: Fetal assessment based upon fetal biophysical profile scoring: Experience in 12,620 referred high risk pregnancies. I. Perinatal mortality by frequency and etiology, *Am J Obstet Gynecol* 151(3):343-350, 1985.

21. Manning FA, Platt LD, Sipos L: Antepartum fetal evaluation: Development of a fetal biophysical profile, *Am J Obstet Gynecol* 13(6):787-795, 1980.

22. Matsuda Y, Takatsugu M, Satoshi K: The critical period of non-reassuring fetal heart rate patterns in preterm gestation, *Eur J Obstet Gynecol Reprod Biol* 106(1):36-39, 2003.

23. Miyazaki FS, Nevarez F: Saline amnioinfusion for relief of repetitive variable decelerations: A prospective randomized study, *Am J Obstet Gynecol* 153(3):301-306, 1985.

24. Miyazaki FS, Taylor NA: Saline amnioinfusion for relief of variable or prolonged decelerations. A preliminary report, *Am J Obstet Gynecol* 146(6):670-678, 1983.

25. Nageotte MP, Bertucci L, Towers CV, Lagrew DL, Modanlou H: Prophylactic amnioinfusion in pregnancies complicated by oligohydramnios: A prospective study, *Obstet Gynecol* 77(5):677-680, 1991.

26. National Institute of Child Health and Human Development Research Planning Workshop: Electronic fetal heart rate monitoring: Research guidelines for interpretation, *Am J Obstet Gynecol* 177(6):1385-1390, 1997.

27. Phelan JP, Smith CV, Broussard P, Small M: Amniotic fluid volume assessment with four-quadrant technique at 36-42 weeks gestation, *J Reprod Med* 32(7):540-542, 1987.

28. Pillai M, James D: The development of fetal heart rate patterns during normal pregnancy, *Obstet Gynecol* 76(5):812-816, 1990.

29. Pollack RN, Hauer-Pollack G, Divon MY: Macrosomia in post-dates pregnancies: The accuracy of routine ultrasonographic screening, *Am J Obstet Gynecol* 167(1):7-11, 1992.

30. Polzin GB, Blakemore KJ, Petrie RH, Amon E: Fetal vibro-acoustic stimulation: Magnitude and duration of fetal heart rate accelerations as a marker of fetal health, *Obstet Gynecol* 72(4):621-626, 1988.

31. Schrimmer DB, Macri CJ, Paul RH: Prophylactic amnioinfusion as a treatment for oligohydramnios in laboring patients: A prospective, randomized trial, *Am J Obstet Gynecol* 165(4 Pt 1):972-975, 1991.

32. Smith CV, Nguyen HN, Phelan JP, Paul RH: Intrapartum assessment of fetal well-being: A comparison of fetal acoustic stimulation with acid-base determinations, *Am J Obstet Gynecol* 155(4):726-728, 1986.

33. Spellacy WN, Miller S, Winegar A, Peterson PQ: Macrosomia—maternal characteristics and infant complications, *Obstet Gynecol* 66(2):158-161, 1985.

34. Usher RH, Boyd ME, McLean FH, Kramer MS: Assessment of fetal risk in postdate pregnancies, *Am J Obstet Gynecol* 158(2):259-264, 1988.

35. Yeh S, Bruce SL, Thorton YS: Intrapartum monitoring and management of the postdate fetus, *Clin Perinatol* 9(2):381-386, 1982.

CHAPTER 8

Fetal Assessment in Non-Obstetric Settings

Assessment and care of the pregnant woman takes place in a variety of settings. Collaboration among perinatal, perioperative, intensive care, and emergency department teams is essential when the pregnant woman is cared for in an area other than the labor and delivery suite. Knowledge of the physiologic and anatomic adaptations of pregnancy is crucial because pregnancy alters anatomy and physiology to such an extent that clinical symptoms may be distorted, and normal discomforts may contribute to a puzzling picture. Some changes are so dramatic that they would be considered pathologic in the nonpregnant woman (Box 8-1). For example, palpation is difficult as the peritoneum stretches to allow displacement of the abdominal organs.

The laboratory values relied on for confirmation of a diagnosis or problem also differ, because of the adaptations required by the body during pregnancy. Furthermore, not only does the pregnant woman present with her unique challenges but she arrives with a fetus who also requires assessment, care, and possible intervention. Fetal stability depends on maternal stability. If caregivers do not understand and support the adaptations of the pregnancy, there is a potential for adverse maternal and fetal events.

The focus of this chapter is to demonstrate the need for collaborative efforts when a pregnant woman requires evaluation. She needs the *right* providers to care for her at the *right* time and in the *right* setting. When she receives care outside of the perinatal unit, it is often because she requires surgical or medical expertise. The needs of the fetus should not be overlooked. The caregivers must have the requisite skills and must be qualified to evaluate the fetus by education, experience, and performance standards. It is imperative that communication between services and providers be clear and timely to ensure that the maternal–fetal dyad receives appropriate care by the most appropriate staff member regardless of the physical setting.

BOX 8-1   Physiologic Adaptations to Pregnancy

Cardiovascular
- Physiologic anemia, hypervolemia (expansion of plasma volume greater than expansion of red cell mass)
- Blood volume increases by 30% to 40% (1200 to 1500 ml higher than prepregnant state)
- Plasma increases 70%, cells 30%
- Hematocrit of 32% to 34% is not unusual
- Cardiac output increases 30% to 50% (a result of increased blood volume)
- Heart rate and stroke volume increase
- Systemic vascular resistance decreases, with resultant decrease in blood pressure and mean arterial pressure
- Uteroplacental vascular bed is dilated; passive low resistance system
- Uterofetoplacental unit receives 20% of cardiac output
- Peripheral edema; dyspnea; presence of third heart sound
- Pelvic venous congestion

Hematologic
- Increased clotting factors VII, VIII, IX, and X, and fibrinogen (hypercoagulable)
- Decreased serum albumin may lower colloid osmotic pressure (predisposing to pulmonary edema)

Renal
- Smooth muscle relaxation, increased urinary stasis, hydronephrosis, hydroureter; increased susceptibility to urinary tract infection
- Increased creatinine clearance
- Decrease in serum creatinine and urea nitrogen (BUN)

Respiratory
- Tidal volume increases by 30% to 40%; respiratory rate unchanged
- Oxygen consumption increases by 20%
- Diaphragm elevated by the growing fetus
- Arterial P_{CO_2} decreases as a result of hyperventilation, resulting in a "compensated" respiratory alkalosis

Gastrointestinal
- Smooth muscle relaxes, increasing gastric emptying time
- Gastric motility decreases, sphincters relax, higher likelihood of aspiration

Musculoskeletal
- Increased risk of ligament injury secondary to relaxin and progesterone
- Shifting center of gravity with growth of fetus, diastasis of the rectus abdominus
- Symphyseal separation

EMERGENCY SERVICES DEPARTMENT ASSESSMENT AND CARE

Pregnant women present to the emergency department (ED) for a variety of reasons. A *primary* survey occurs at triage: "Why are you here?" A *secondary* survey includes obtaining information about signs, symptoms, the mechanism of injury, and evaluation of pain. This is, of course, predicated on the woman's ability to communicate and the absence of trauma that would prevent communication.

Findings from the primary survey and identification of gestational age are usually the best indicators for the unit in which the woman's care would be most appropriately managed. Special attention to the pregnancy is a part of the assessment and not merely an afterthought. Before discharge from the emergency department or transfer to another area, assessment to confirm both maternal *and* fetal well-being is required. *Where* the assessment takes place is not the concern. Rather, it is *who* is performing the assessment and whether the person is qualified by virtue of education and competency in obstetrics.

Women present to an emergency unit for numerous nonpregnancy- and pregnancy-related reasons. Many emergency units use 20 weeks of gestation as a determinant of whether care should be managed in the emergency department or in labor and delivery. Women who present to the emergency department at a gestation of more than 20 weeks complaining of well-recognized obstetric concerns (e.g., vaginal bleeding, contractions, rupture of membranes, increased or watery vaginal discharge, abdominal pain, pelvic pressure, decreased fetal movement) may be transferred immediately to the labor and delivery unit for further assessment and management. For those women with vague symptoms, such as headache, edema, nausea and vomiting, or "just not feeling well," the decision about where to evaluate is not always so clear. These vague symptoms may be associated with the hypertensive disorders of pregnancy, such as preeclampsia or HELLP syndrome (characterized by hemolysis [H], elevated liver [EL] enzymes, and low platelets [LP]). Well-meaning care in a non-obstetric setting for the woman with a hypertensive disorder of pregnancy has the potential of being detrimental to both the woman and the fetus. Alternatively, these vague symptoms could reflect influenza, food poisoning, cholecystitis, or migraine headaches. A telephone discussion between the emergency department and the labor and delivery unit may be the best method of determining whose expertise is most needed for the evaluation and care of the maternal–fetal dyad.

When a woman of more than 20 weeks of gestation presents to the emergency department with cardiovascular, respiratory, or orthopedic complaints, the maternal and fetal vital signs should be assessed and documented. Appropriate emergency department screening questions, regardless of the reason she presents for triage, include the following:

- Is your baby's movement today the same as in previous days?
- Are you having any cramping, pelvic pressure, backache, or contractions?
- Is there any vaginal bleeding or leaking of fluid?

A decision tree is useful for triage of the maternal–fetal dyad. Although emergency department staff may have algorithms to follow for geriatric, pediatric, and nonpregnant adult patients, standard algorithms specific for the pregnant woman are uncommon. Some facilities develop their own written guidelines for appropriate care. To consistently meet the standards of care for a pregnant woman who presents to the facility for any reason, a triage decision tree should be developed by the emergency department and obstetric staff. The triage decision tree should be used to determine whether the woman should remain in the emergency department or be transferred to surgery, critical care, or the labor and delivery suite (Figure 8-1).

The following chart is an example of a brief decision guide:

Woman of less than 20 weeks of gestation, regardless of concern	Emergency services department
Woman of more than 20 weeks of gestation with a pregnancy-related concern	Labor and delivery
Woman of more than 20 weeks of gestation with a nonpregnancy-related issue	ED with obstetric consult

The term *obstetric consultation* requires definition by each institution. It may mean fetal assessment or monitoring in the emergency department by an emergency department registered nurse who is competent in obstetrics, or it could mean that a labor and delivery nurse or obstetric provider goes to the emergency department to evaluate the woman. Another option is to provide care in the emergency department and then transfer the woman to the labor and delivery unit for assessment. Furthermore, *pregnancy-related* may be difficult to define. The fetus may be best served by having a labor and delivery caregiver evaluate the woman in the emergency department so that the woman and fetus are cared for simultaneously. This approach becomes more significant when trauma is involved.

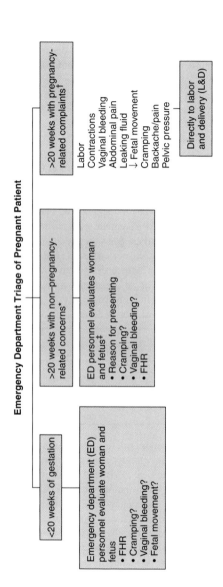

Emergency Department Triage of Pregnant Patient

<20 weeks of gestation

Emergency department (ED) personnel evaluate woman and fetus
• FHR
• Cramping?
• Vaginal bleeding?
• Fetal movement

>20 weeks with non–pregnancy-related concerns*

ED personnel evaluates woman and fetus‡
• Reason for presenting
• Cramping?
• Vaginal bleeding?
• FHR

>20 weeks with pregnancy-related complaints†

Labor
Contractions
Vaginal bleeding
Abdominal pain
Leaking fluid
↓ Fetal movement
Cramping
Backache/pain
Pelvic pressure

Directly to labor and delivery (L&D)

*When a woman at >20 weeks of gestation arrives at the ED with an *emergency* medical condition (e.g., trauma), she is evaluated in the ED immediately, and the L&D nurse is called to come to the ED to assess and monitor the fetus and the pregnancy.
†The pregnant woman may present with headache, nausea and vomiting, epigastric pain, or visual changes, and these may be pregnancy related.
‡ED physician may ask L&D nurse to come to the ED for fetal monitoring when gestation is >24 weeks, *or* the pregnant woman may be sent to L&D triage for fetal assessment after being seen by the ED physician. L&D nurse reports triage assessment to obstetrician.

FIGURE 8-1 ED triage of pregnant patient.

A helpful tool for establishing institutional guidelines is *The Obstetrical Patient in the ED,* a joint position statement by the Emergency Nurses Association (ENA) and the Association of Women's Health, Obstetric and Neonatal Nurses (AWHONN). Initiated in 1988, the statement has been revised[8] and can be located on the ENA website at www.ena.org.

PREGNANT TRAUMA VICTIM ASSESSMENT AND CARE

Trauma is the leading cause of death in women of childbearing years, and it is the highest non-obstetric cause of death during pregnancy. Trauma occurring in pregnancy is complicated. Trauma teams are often not accustomed to caring for pregnant women and their physiologic adaptations specific to gestation, and obstetric teams are unfamiliar with caring for trauma patients. Certain injuries are unique to the pregnant trauma patient: uterine damage, placental abruption, and intrauterine fetal demise. Consideration of gestational age is an important factor. A decision must be made about the willingness to intervene operatively on behalf of the fetus. In addition, the impact of maternal trauma on the fetus may not be immediate. When there has been blunt abdominal trauma or when vaginal bleeding is present, the blood must be examined for fetal blood and the fetus monitored over several hours. It is inadequate in this situation to be reassured by a normal fetal heart rate (FHR) tracing. Trauma concerns specific to pregnancy are in Table 8-1.

The *primary survey* of an injured pregnant woman addresses the same concerns, such as the ABCs (airway, breathing, circulation) addressed for any other trauma victim, with the woman receiving priority over the fetus. Supplemental oxygen may be essential to prevent both maternal and fetal hypoxemia. Survival of the fetus depends on adequate uterine perfusion and the delivery of oxygen. Catecholamine release due to either anxiety or hemorrhage can cause uteroplacental vasoconstriction and can compromise fetal circulation. Avoiding the supine position optimizes maternal and fetal hemodynamics. Uterine blood flow represents 10% to 15% of maternal cardiac output, or approximately 700 to 800 ml per minute. Diversion of blood flow from the uterus to maternal vital organs from hypovolemia may, depending on severity and duration, eventually lead to fetal tachycardia, decreased variability, and late decelerations, *even before* there are changes

TABLE 8-1   Trauma Concerns Specific to Pregnancy

Abruption	
Result of "shearing" effect when uterus is deformed by external forces, causing separation from placenta	Can trigger diffuse intravascular coagulation because of high concentration of thromboplastin in placenta
	Electronic fetal monitoring is most sensitive means of detecting abruption
	Ultrasound most specific but lacks sensitivity
Vaginal bleeding poor predictor of abruption	May be a later sign; watch for increasing fundal height, increased uterine activity, increased pain
Uterine Rupture	
Blunt trauma	Use ultrasound, x-ray; palpate fetal parts outside uterus; assess pain
Maternal–Fetal Hemorrhage	
Four to five times more common in injured woman than in noninjured woman	Fetal anemia, death, or isoimmunization
Fetal Compromise	
Nonspecific complication but most common	Late decelerations, tachycardia, loss of variability
Preterm Contractions	
Common after blunt trauma	Abruption with potential for fetal hypoxia
Fetal Injuries	
Skull fractures, intracranial hemorrhage	More common in third trimester

in maternal vital signs. Thus aggressive volume resuscitation is encouraged even when the hypovolemic woman is normotensive. The fetus can act as an internal pulse oximeter for the woman, as evidenced by fetal heart rate patterns that reflect fetal hypoxemia secondary to maternal hypovolemia and reduced uteroplacental perfusion.

Emergency management of the pregnant trauma victim summarized by Kass and Abbott[11] involves the following:

- Maternal resuscitation (emergency cesarean delivery at more than 24 weeks may be indicated to facilitate resuscitation in maternal arrest)
- Optimization of maternal oxygenation

- Optimization of intravascular volume
- Prevention or treatment of supine hypotension
- Avoid hesitation about needed radiographic imaging
- Intubate early if not oxygenating well
- Abdominal ultrasound evaluation for retroperitoneal hemorrhage
- Determination of fetal cardiac activity and gestational age
- Obstetric consultation immediately after primary survey
- Electronic fetal monitoring when fetus is more than 24 weeks of gestation
- Immune globulin (RhoGAM) to all Rh-negative women who are known to be unsensitized

The *secondary survey* or assessment involves performing a physical examination, evaluating the pregnancy, and monitoring the fetus. The obstetric history should cover the following:

- Last menstrual period and estimated date of delivery or of confinement
- Problems and complications of the pregnancy
- Measurement of fundal height to approximate gestational age
- Presence of vaginal bleeding
- Evaluation for ruptured membranes
- Uterine activity
- Fetal activity and movement
- Assessment of placenta for placental abruption with ultrasound
- A Kleihauer-Betke test from maternal blood to evaluate for fetal-maternal hemorrhage

Fetal evaluation begins with an assessment of fetal movement and fetal heart rate. Doppler ultrasound may be used initially to locate and assess the fetal heart rate. Then, electronic fetal monitoring remains the most valuable adjunct tool for fetal evaluation in the gestation that is greater than 24 weeks. Electronic monitoring of the fetus and evaluation of uterine activity are integral parts of the early and ongoing assessment of the fetus, as they allow early recognition of the response to volume therapy or of sudden deterioration of fetal status. In addition, uterine irritability or contractions palpated or observed on the tracing may provide clues to placental abruption, trauma, or uterine injury. Loss of variability and late or prolonged decelerations are the most sensitive findings in the detection of abruption.[1] Bedside ultrasonography can be useful to detect fetal cardiac activity and to measure amniotic fluid volume. Although the sensitivity for abruption is not good, ultrasound may help identify and evaluate changes in subchorionic bleeding.

The Kleihauer-Betke test can estimate the volume of fetal blood in the maternal circulation but cannot predict other complications. It should not replace fetal monitoring and ultrasound.[11] This test may be helpful in determining the amount of RhoGAM needed for the unsensitized Rh-negative woman experiencing trauma, but it should not be used to determine the *need* for RhoGAM. If significant fetal hemorrhage has occurred, it is likely to manifest in the fetal heart rate tracing as fetal tachycardia and decreased variability. Fetal heart rate changes indicative of hypoxemia combined with a positive Kleihauer-Betke may signal fetal anemia and potential fetal compromise.

During maternal hypovolemia the maternal circulation is protected at the expense of uterine perfusion. Maternal hypotension occurs relatively late in the progression of hypovolemic shock, after more than 30% of the maternal circulating volume has been lost. The vasoconstrictive effects of maternal hypoxia, acidosis, and sympathetic stimulation are often seen in hypovolemic shock and can compromise uterine perfusion and fetal oxygenation. Adequate fluid resuscitation is imperative to maintain uterine perfusion and protect the fetus. The fetal heart rate tracing is a valuable tool for reflecting maternal cardiovascular and respiratory well-being.

There are *two indications for an emergent cesarean delivery*:

1. deteriorating status of a viable fetus despite resuscitative efforts, and
2. a moribund woman who does not respond to initial primary interventions of trauma resuscitation.[13]

As in cardiac arrest, delivery of the fetus may allow not only fetal resuscitation but also restoration of maternal venous return and perhaps a successful maternal resuscitation. A decision tree for the unstable pregnant trauma patient may be a useful resource (Figure 8-2).

Once stabilized, a woman with trauma can often be transferred to the perinatal unit for continued care and monitoring. If she remains unstable, she may need to be transferred to surgery or to the intensive or critical care unit. The intrapartum or labor and delivery nurse should continue caring for the pregnant woman and her fetus regardless of where the woman has been transferred. Again, where the assessment and care take place is not the concern. What is important is that the individual who is performing and interpreting information is the most competent person to do so.

Electronic fetal monitoring should be used for fetal and uterine assessment after trauma; however, there are no well-established

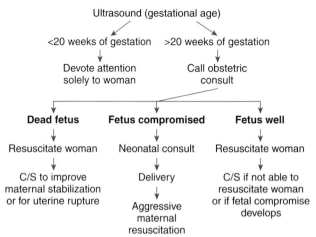

FIGURE 8-2 Decision tree for the pregnant woman who is unstable after trauma. *C/S*, Cesarean section.

standards for the duration.[3,5] Many centers advocate 24 hours of continuous fetal monitoring. However, numerous studies have been done to determine risks that predict a poor outcome so that guidelines for electronic monitoring can be established.[4,16] A pregnant woman who has sustained blunt abdominal trauma with any risk factors for preterm labor or abruption should be monitored up to 24 hours. Those without these risk factors can safely be monitored for 6 hours and then discharged.[6] If the fetus appears healthy on initial evaluation, frequent uterine contractions (more than eight per hour) in the first 4 hours is a sensitive, if nonspecific, predictor of later fetal complications and mandates a longer period of assessment. If the woman has no contractions or bleeding, and there is evidence of fetal movement on the fetal monitor tracing with reassuring parameters, 4 hours is probably a long enough evaluation period.[1] It is imperative to establish a baseline fetal heart rate, and any fetal tachycardia should be regarded with considerable suspicion. At discharge, the signs and symptoms of preterm labor along with the procedure for performing daily fetal kick counts should be reviewed with the woman, and she should be given instructions for when to notify the health care provider.

Safety during pregnancy should be discussed before discharging a pregnant woman from the emergency department or the labor and delivery unit. Anatomic adaptations to pregnancy are associated with problems with coordination and balance, and falls are more common. Discussing safety features, proper body mechanics, and the avoidance of toxic chemicals may help the pregnant woman to avoid accidents. Instruction about appropriate seat belt use during pregnancy is an important aspect of discharge education. A combination lap belt and shoulder harness is the most effective auto restraint, and both should be used. The lap belt is worn low, underneath the uterus, and as snug as is comfortable. The shoulder harness is worn above the uterus and below the neck. The headrest can also prevent whiplash.[7,15]

MATERNAL–FETAL TRANSPORT ASSESSMENT AND CARE

First responders must understand the concepts presented in this chapter to provide appropriate care. It is vital that the emergency medical technician, paramedic, and firefighter personnel promote maternal circulation and oxygenation and consider occult hemorrhage and shock in the pregnant trauma victim. All pregnant women should have supplemental oxygen and intravenous access established en route to the emergency department. Alerting the hospital early during transport allows the staff to inform the obstetric staff of the need for collaborative care immediately upon arrival. These first responders must understand the importance of transporting a pregnant woman of more than 20 weeks of gestation on her side or with a backboard tilt of 15 degrees to prevent supine hypotension.[11] Information regarding uterine status should be obtained, and the woman should be asked about fetal activity. Vital signs should be assessed as often as they are for the nonpregnant woman, and uterine and fetal status should be evaluated whenever possible. Fundal height determination may be of great benefit in determining fetal age and the need for prompt obstetric intervention on arrival to the emergency department. Simply noting the height of the uterus as above or below the maternal umbilicus may help determine if the pregnancy is more than or less than 20 weeks of gestation.

NON-OBSTETRIC SURGERY: MATERNAL–FETAL ASSESSMENT AND CARE

It is estimated that 50,000 gravid women each year have surgery during their pregnancy.[10,12] The key points for caring for this dyad during surgery are collaboration and communication with all team members. During surgery, the goals for intact fetal survival include the following:

- Maintaining maternal blood pressure
- Maintaining maternal oxygenation
- Maintaining maternal circulating volume

A standard of care does not exist for assessing the fetus during non-obstetric procedures or for intervening on behalf of the fetus at early (less than 24 weeks) gestation. In fact, conflicting expert opinions exist regarding the necessity of intraoperative monitoring.[9,10] Decisions based on clinical context are key. As the American College of Obstetricians and Gynecologists states, "The decision to use fetal monitoring should be individualized and, if used, may be based on gestational age, type of surgery, and facilities available."[2] The advantages of monitoring for surgical procedures include enhanced communication among disciplines to focus on the safety of drugs for the fetus, patient positioning with regard to the effects on the fetus, altered maternal anatomy and physiology due to pregnancy, and the identification and need for an emergent cesarean delivery. Abdominal surgery commonly results in preterm contractions, which may evolve into preterm labor and birth. Thus providers often consider administration of tocolytic agents before and after surgical procedures, especially abdominal procedures, that are likely to stimulate uterine activity.[10] These surgeries include placement of a renal stent, appendectomy, cholecystectomy, ovarian cyst and tumor removal, and trauma. Collaboration among the surgeon, anesthesiologist, and obstetrician ensures the safety of both patients and determines if intraoperative fetal assessment is necessary. Alerting the neonatal staff when the fetus is viable is also important for timely care for both patients.

SURGERY WHEN GESTATION IS MORE THAN 24 WEEKS

When surgery is needed by a woman whose gestation is more than 24 weeks, the following points should be kept in mind:

- Preoperative cervical examination provides baseline information.
- Preoperative administration of a tocolytic medication such as Indocin may help prevent preterm contractions and uterine irritability.
- Preoperative medications are indicated to assist with gastric emptying and neutralizing gastric content, because of decreased gastric motility and relaxed gastric sphincters.

- Left uterine displacement after 20 weeks of gestation assists in avoiding hypotension and providing improved uteroplacental perfusion.
- Maintaining maternal oxygen saturation above 95% and maternal mean arterial pressure greater than 65 mm Hg helps keep the uterus perfused.
- Preoperative monitoring of the gravid uterus in a pregnancy of more than 24 weeks of gestation should be done with equipment appropriate for gestational age and by a clinician who is adept at both performing the procedure and interpreting the status of uterine activity and FHR patterns.
- Intraoperative monitoring (at >24 weeks) can be done with a Doppler or an ultrasound transducer (covered with a sterile sleeve). Interpretation and management of intraoperative FHR changes should be guided by the principles outlined in Chapters 2, 5, and 6.
- Postoperative monitoring of uterine activity and fetal assessment in the postanesthesia care unit are continued as appropriate for gestational age, type of surgery performed, obstetrician's orders, and the presence or absence of uterine contractions.
- Surgery during pregnancy brings with it the risk of an urgent cesarean delivery. The neonatal staff should be notified and available for any neonatal emergencies that might arise. Depending on the surgery, an obstetrician may be present at the surgery or at least informed that the procedure is being performed.[10]

The multidisciplinary approach to the pregnant surgical patient is optimal. Formulating a perioperative plan of care enhances the outcome for the maternal–fetal dyad. Communication among, and involvement of, all team members ensures the best possible outcome.

FEDERAL LAW AND TRIAGE

Triage incorporates a rapid assessment of the woman, identification of the concerns, determination of the acuity of the problem, and arrangement for the appropriate personnel and equipment to meet the woman's needs. Triage of all perinatal women is regulated by federal law via the Emergency Medical Treatment and Active Labor Act (EMTALA). This act requires that all hospitals provide a medical screening examination to determine if an emergency medical condition exists or if a woman is in labor. Prompt triage and a medical screening examination (MSE) must be performed in a timely manner, and if an emergency situation exists, treatment and stabilization are required prior to discharge or transfer.[14] The ENA and AWHONN support the development of hospital policies and procedures that specifically outline triage, care, and disposition of the pregnant woman. Their position statement referred to earlier in the chapter states that the care of a woman should take place in the area best prepared to handle her needs.[8]

SUMMARY

The initial emergent event and the physiologic challenges of pregnant women require exceptional teamwork and communication, combined with workable institutional protocols. Caregivers in the emergency department should understand fetal and maternal physiology to provide safe care to pregnant women. Collaboration between the emergency department and the labor and delivery staff is essential for developing guidelines and protocols.

References

1. Abbott J: Emergency management of the obstetric patient. In Burrow G, Duffy T, editors: *Medical complications during pregnancy*, ed 5, Philadelphia, 1999, Saunders.
2. American College of Obstetricians and Gynecologists: Non-obstetric surgery in pregnancy, *Committee Opinion* no. 284, Washington, DC, 2003, ACOG.
3. American College of Obstetricians and Gynecologists: Obstetric aspects of management: Trauma, *Educational Bulletin* no. 251, Washington, DC, 1998, ACOG.
4. Biester E, Tomich P, Esposito T, Weber L: Trauma in pregnancy: Normal revised trauma score in relation to other markers of maternofetal status: A preliminary study, *Am J Obstet Gynecol* 176(6):1206-1212, 1997.
5. Colburn V: Trauma in pregnancy, *J Perinat Neonatal Nurs* 13(3):21-32, 1999.
6. Curet M, Schermer CR, Demarest GB, Bieneik EJ 3rd, Curet LB: Predictors of outcome in trauma during pregnancy: Identification of patients who can be monitored for less than 6 hours, *J Trauma* 49(1):18-25, 2000.
7. Dobo S, Johnson V: Evaluation and care of the pregnant patient with minor trauma, *Clin Fam Pract* 2(3):707-722, 2000.
8. Emergency Nurses Association, Association of Women's Health, Obstetric and Neonatal Nurses: *Joint position statement: The obstetrical patient in the ED*, Des Plaines, IL, 2000, ENA.

9. Horrigan T, Villareal R, Weinstein L: Are obstetrical personnel required for intraoperative fetal monitoring during non-obstetrical surgery? *J Perinatol* 19(2):124-126, 1999.

10. Inturrisi M: Perioperative assessment of fetal heart rate and uterine activity, *J Obstet Gynecol Neonatal Nurs* 29(3):331-336, 2000.

11. Kass L, Abbot J: Trauma in pregnancy. In Ferrera PC, Colucciello SA, Verdile V, Marx A, editors: *Trauma management: An emergency medicine approach,* St Louis, 2001, Mosby.

12. Kendrick JM, Powers PH: Perioperative care of the pregnant surgical patient, *AORN J* 60(2):205-216, 1994.

13. Luppi C: Cardiopulmonary resuscitation in pregnancy. In Mandeville LK, Troino NH, editors: *High-risk and critical care: Intrapartum nursing*, ed 2, Philadelphia, 1999, Lippincott Williams & Wilkins.

14. Mahlmeister L, Van Mullem C: The process of triage in perinatal settings: Clinical and legal issues, *J Perinat Neonatal Nurs* 13(4):13-30, 2000.

15. Saunders R: Nursing care during pregnancy. In Lowdermilk DL, Perry SE, editors: *Maternity & women's health care*, ed 8, St Louis, 2004, Mosby.

16. Shah K, Simons RK, Holbrook T, Fortlage D, Winchell RJ, Hoyt DB: Trauma in pregnancy: Maternal and fetal outcomes, *J Trauma* 45(1):83-86, 1998.

Bibliography

Blackburn, ST: *Maternal, fetal, & neonatal physiology: A clinical perspective*, ed 3, St. Louis, 2007, Saunders.

Daddario J: Trauma in pregnancy. In Mandeville L, Troiano N, editors: *High-risk and critical care: Intrapartum nursing*, ed 2, Philadelphia, 1999, Lippincott, Williams & Wilkins.

Jevon P, Raby M, O'Donnell E: *Resuscitation in pregnancy: A practical approach*, Oxford, 2001, Butterworth Heinemann.

Johnson M, Luppi C, Over D: Cardiopulmonary resuscitation. In Gambling D, Douglas MJ, editors: *Obstetric anesthesia and common disorders*, Philadelphia, 1999, Saunders.

Kendrick JM: Fetal and uterine response during maternal surgery, *MCN Am J Matern Child Nurs* 19(3):165-170, 1994.

Kendrick JM, Woodard CB, Cross SB: Surveyed use of fetal and uterine monitoring during maternal surgery, *AORN J* 62(3):386-392, 1995.

Simpson KR: Critical illness during pregnancy: considerations for evaluation and treatment of the fetus as the second patient, *Crit Care Nurs Q* 29(1): 20-31, 2006.

Simpson KR: Fetal assessment in the adult intensive care unit, *Crit Care Nurs Clin North Am* 16(2):233-242, 2004.

Antepartum Fetal Assessment

Early in its development, electronic fetal heart rate (FHR) monitoring required direct access to the fetus and was limited to the intrapartum period. Later, Doppler ultrasound technology made it possible to monitor the fetal heart rate before labor. The experience gained from intrapartum monitoring was applied to the antepartum period and led to the development of antepartum testing.

The goals of antepartum testing are the following:

1. To identify fetuses at risk for injury due to disrupted oxygenation so that permanent injury or death might be prevented
2. To identify healthy fetuses so that unnecessary intervention can be avoided

FUNDAMENTAL DETERMINATIONS

The key measure of the effectiveness of an antepartum test is the *false-negative rate*, defined most often in the literature as the incidence of fetal death within 1 week of a normal antepartum test. Reported false-negative rates range from 0.4 to 1.9 per 1000 with current testing methods.

Another important measure is the false-positive rate. A *false-positive test* is usually defined as an abnormal test that prompts delivery but that is not associated with evidence of acute disruption of fetal oxygenation (meconium-stained amniotic fluid, intrapartum "fetal distress," or low Apgar scores) or chronic disruption of fetal oxygenation (fetal growth restriction under the 10th percentile for gestational age). False-positive rates range from 30% to 90% with current testing methods (Box 9-1).

Antepartum testing is used primarily in patients who are considered to be at increased risk for disrupted fetal oxygenation. The optimal gestational age at which to begin antepartum testing is not known. However, for most medical indications, testing is initiated by 32 to 34 weeks. The usual timing of antepartum testing for obstetric indications is described in Table 9-1. Initiating testing prior to 32 weeks might be expected to prevent more fetal deaths. However, fetal death resulting from disrupted oxygenation is uncommon prior to 32 to 34 weeks.

BOX 9-1 Key Measures of the Effectiveness of Antepartum Testing

False negative: Fetal death within 1 week of a normal antepartum test
False positive: Abnormal test that prompts delivery but is not
  associated with acute or chronic disruption of fetal oxygenation

TABLE 9-1 Timing of Initiation of Antepartum Testing for Obstetric Indications

Obstetric Indications	Medical Indications
Postterm pregnancy	40–41 weeks
Unexplained elevated AFP, hCG	32–34 weeks
Cholestasis of pregnancy	32–34 weeks
Antiphospholipid syndrome	32–34 weeks
Previous unexplained stillbirth	32–34 weeks*
Suspected fetal growth restriction	At diagnosis
Decreased fetal movement	At diagnosis
Preeclampsia	At diagnosis
Multiple gestation (discordant)	At diagnosis
Alloimmunization	At diagnosis
Oligohydramnios	At diagnosis

*Or one week earlier than previous loss
AFP, alpha fetoprotein; hCG, human chorionic gonadotropin.

Moreover, in view of the high false-positive rates of most testing protocols, earlier initiation of testing should be expected to increase the incidence of unnecessary intervention and iatrogenic prematurity, with its attendant complications.

Indications for Antepartum Testing

Common obstetric and medical indications for antepartum testing are as follows:

Obstetric Indications
- Postterm pregnancy
- Unexplained elevated alpha fetoprotein (AFP), human chorionic gonadotropin (hCG)
- Cholestasis of pregnancy
- Antiphospholipid antibody syndrome
- Previous unexplained stillbirth
- Suspected fetal growth restriction
- Decreased fetal movement
- Preeclampsia
- Multiple gestation (discordant)

Obstetric Indications (Cont'd.)
- Alloimmunization
- Oligohydramnios

Medical Indications
- Diabetes
- Chronic hypertension
- Cyanotic cardiac disease
- Renal disease
- Thyroid disease
- Collagen vascular disease
- Substance abuse
- Pulmonary disease (severe asthma)
- Hemoglobinopathy

CONTRACTION STRESS TEST AND OXYTOCIN CHALLENGE TEST

The first antepartum testing technique, the contraction stress test or oxytocin challenge test, arose from intrapartum observations linking late decelerations with poor perinatal outcome. The test sought to identify transient fetal hypoxemia by demonstrating late decelerations in fetuses exposed to the stress of spontaneous (contraction stress test) or induced (oxytocin challenge test) uterine contractions. Kubli and associates found that late decelerations occurring during spontaneous uterine contractions were associated with increased rates of fetal death, growth retardation, and neonatal depression.[14] Similar observations were made by other investigators using oxytocin or nipple stimulation to provoke uterine contractions.

Interpretation and Management

The contraction stress test is considered *negative* if there are at least three uterine contractions in a 10-minute period with no late decelerations on the tracing. In this case, the routine weekly testing schedule is resumed. Failure to produce three contractions within a 10-minute window, or inability to trace the fetal heart rate, results in an *unsatisfactory* test. Prolonged decelerations, variable decelerations, or late decelerations occurring with less than 50% of the contractions constitute a *suspicious or equivocal* test. Decelerations that occur in the presence of contractions more frequent than every 2 minutes or lasting longer than 90 seconds constitute an *equivocal-hyperstimulatory* test. Unsatisfactory, suspicious, or equivocal tests require repeat testing the following day.

The contraction stress test or oxytocin challenge test is considered *positive* when at least half of the contractions during a 10-minute window are associated with late decelerations. Usually, a positive contraction stress test or oxytocin challenge test warrants hospitalization for further evaluation and/or delivery. Freeman and colleagues tested more than 4600 women with the contraction stress test and reported a false-negative rate of 0.4/1000.[10] When the last test before delivery was a negative contraction stress test, the perinatal mortality rate was 2.3/1000, compared to a mortality rate of 176.5/1000 when the last test was a positive contraction stress test. Reported false-positive rates for the contraction stress test range from 8% to 57% with an average of approximately 30%.[15]

Interpretation summary of the contraction stress test is as follows:

- Negative: No late or significant variable decelerations
- Positive: Late decelerations with 50% or more of contractions (even if there are fewer than three contractions in 10 minutes)
- Equivocal-suspicious: Intermittent late decelerations or significant variable decelerations
- Equivocal-hyperstimulatory: Fetal heart rate decelerations that occur in the presence of contractions more frequently than every 2 minutes or lasting longer than 90 seconds
- Unsatisfactory: Fewer than three contractions in 10 minutes *or* an uninterpretable tracing

Advantages and Limitations

Principal *advantages* of the contraction stress test include excellent sensitivity and a weekly testing interval. *Limitations* include a high rate of equivocal results requiring repeat testing, increased expense and inconvenience (particularly if oxytocin is required), and increased time requirement compared to the nonstress test.

Procedures for Contraction Stress Testing

The contraction stress test can be performed by breast or nipple stimulation or by administering an intravenous infusion with oxytocin. Note that the *contraction stress test is contraindicated* in several clinical situations, including preterm labor, placenta previa, vasa previa, cervical incompetence, multiple gestation, and previous classical cesarean section. The procedure for performing the contraction stress test follows.

Procedure for Nipple-Stimulated Contraction Stress Test

1. Assist the woman to a semi-Fowler's position with a lateral tilt.
2. Position the tocodynamometer above the uterine fundus.
3. Place the ultrasound transducer on the maternal abdomen where the clearest fetal signal can be obtained.
4. Monitor baseline FHR and uterine activity until 10 minutes of interpretable data are obtained (defer nipple stimulation if three spontaneous unstimulated contractions of more than 40 seconds' duration occur within a 10-minute period).
5. Instruct woman to brush palmar surface of the fingers over the nipple of one breast through her clothes; continue four cycles of 2 minutes on and 2 to 5 minutes off; stop when contraction begins and restimulate when contraction ends (if a 2-minute period has elapsed).
   a. If unsuccessful after four cycles, restimulate the breasts for 10 minutes, stopping when contraction begins and resuming when contraction ends.
   b. If unsuccessful, begin bilateral continuous stimulation for 10 minutes, stopping when contraction begins and resuming when contraction ends.
6. Discontinue nipple stimulation when three or more spontaneous contractions lasting longer than 40 seconds occur in a 10-minute period and are palpable to the examiner.
7. Interpret results and continue monitoring until uterine activity has returned to the prestimulation state.

If nipple stimulation does not produce the desired uterine activity, an oxytocin-stimulated contraction stress test may be necessary.

Procedure for Oxytocin Challenge Test

The oxytocin challenge test is performed in the inpatient setting because labor may be stimulated in some sensitive women, particularly in those at term.

1. Assist the woman into a semi-Fowler's position with a lateral tilt.
2. Place the tocodynamometer above the uterine fundus.
3. Place the ultrasound transducer where the clearest fetal heart sound can be heard—usually below the umbilicus.
4. Monitor baseline FHR and uterine activity until 10 minutes of interpretable data are obtained before administration of oxytocin.

5. Check the woman's blood pressure and pulse (following facility policy).
6. If fewer than three spontaneous unstimulated contractions occur within a 10-minute period and if late decelerations do not occur with spontaneous contractions, oxytocin can be initiated.
7. Piggyback oxytocin into the primary intravenous line in the port nearest the intravenous insertion site.
8. Administer oxytocin, beginning with 0.5 to 2.0 mU/min, with a constant infusion pump per facility protocol.
9. Increase the dosage of oxytocin infusion by 0.5 to 1.0 mU/min at 15-minute intervals until the contraction frequency is three in 10 minutes of 40 seconds' or more duration and contractions are palpable to the examiner.
10. Discontinue the oxytocin when three contractions have occurred within a 10-minute period of interpretable data.
11. Discontinue the oxytocin any time there is evidence of excessive uterine activity, prolonged deceleration, or recurrent late decelerations; be prepared to administer terbutaline for tocolysis.
12. Continue to monitor until uterine activity and FHR return to baseline status.

THE NONSTRESS TEST

Fetal heart rate accelerations that occur in association with fetal movements form the basis of the nonstress test (NST). Although many criteria have been reported, a normal or "reactive" nonstress test usually is defined by two accelerations in a 20-minute period, each lasting at least 15 seconds and peaking at least 15 beats per minute (bpm) above the baseline. Before 32 weeks, an acceleration is defined as a rise of at least 10 bpm with an onset to offset of at least 10 seconds.[2,31]

In most institutions, the test is repeated once or twice weekly. Boehm reported that the latter approach yielded a threefold reduction in the incidence of fetal death.[4] As discussed in Chapter 6, a fetal heart rate acceleration in response to fetal vibroacoustic stimulation is highly predictive of normal fetal pH.* If the fetal heart rate tracing is not spontaneously reactive, vibroacoustic stimulation can be performed by placing an artificial larynx on the maternal abdomen over the fetal head continuously for 1 to 5 seconds.

---

*References 5,6,8,9,12,37-40.

Among 1542 women tested weekly with the nonstress test, Freeman reported a corrected fetal loss rate of 3.2/1000 and a false-negative rate of 1.9/1000.[10] Manning and colleagues reported an average false-negative rate of 6.4/1000 among nine large clinical trials using the nonstress test as the primary method of surveillance.[17] Assessment of fetal heart rate characteristics other than reactivity (baseline rate, variability, decelerations) may improve the sensitivity of the test. Decelerations may be observed in 33% to 50% patients undergoing weekly nonstress tests.[27,35,36] In one study, reactive tests accompanied by variable decelerations were associated with rates of meconium passage and cesarean delivery for fetal indications that were similar to those encountered with nonreactive tests.[35] Manning and colleagues concluded that fetal heart rate decelerations during the nonstress test, regardless of reactivity, warrant consideration of delivery. Reported false-positive rates of the nonstress test vary widely, with an average rate of approximately 50%.

Interpretation and Management

The nonstress test is interpreted as reactive or nonreactive.

- A *reactive* NST is defined as two accelerations in a 20-minute period, each lasting at least 15 seconds and peaking at least 15 bpm above the baseline. (Before 32 weeks an acceleration is defined as a rise of at least 10 bpm lasting at least 10 seconds from onset to offset).
- A *nonreactive* NST is a test that does not demonstrate at least two qualifying accelerations within a 20-minute window.

A reactive nonstress test with no significant decelerations is considered a normal test, and the routine testing schedule is resumed (usually once or twice weekly). A nonreactive nonstress test requires further evaluation. In most cases, a back-up test is performed (a contraction stress test, or more commonly, a biophysical profile). Management is guided by the results of the back-up test. When performed twice weekly and interpreted in the context of associated fetal heart rate patterns, the nonstress test alone appears to be an acceptable, though not optimal, method of antepartum testing.

Advantages and Disadvantages

Advantages of the nonstress test include ease of use and interpretation, low cost, and minimal time requirement. The chief *disadvantages* include a twice-weekly testing interval, a high false-positive rate,

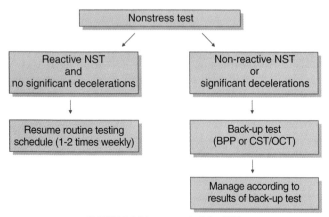

FIGURE 9-1 Management of the NST.

and a higher false-negative rate than achieved with other methods. Management of the nonstress test is illustrated in Figure 9-1.

THE BIOPHYSICAL PROFILE

The biophysical profile, as described by Manning and colleagues,[20] assesses five biophysical variables. Fetal heart rate reactivity, fetal movement, tone, and breathing reflect acute central nervous system function, while amniotic fluid volume serves as a marker of the longer-term adequacy of placental function. Two points are assigned for each normal variable and zero points for each abnormal variable, for a maximum score of 10.

Interpretation and Management

Scoring the biophysical profile:

Biophysical Variable	Normal (Score = 2)	Abnormal (Score = 0)
Fetal breathing movements	At least one episode of fetal breathing movements of at least 30-second duration in a 30-minute observation	Absent fetal breathing movements or less than 30 seconds of sustained fetal breathing movements in 30 minutes

Biophysical Variable	Normal (Score = 2)	Abnormal (Score = 0)
Fetal movements	At least three trunk/limb movements in 30 minutes	Fewer than three episodes of trunk/limb movements in 30 minutes
Fetal tone	At least one episode of active extension with return to flexion of fetal limb or trunk; opening and closing of hand considered normal tone	Absence of movement or slow extension/flexion
Amniotic fluid index (AFI)	AFI >5 cm or at least one pocket >2 cm	AFI ≤5 cm and no single pocket >2 cm
NST	Reactive	Nonreactive

A biophysical profile score of 8 to 10, with normal amniotic fluid volume, is considered normal, and the routine testing schedule is resumed. A score of 6 is considered suspicious, and testing is usually repeated the following day. Scores less than 6 are associated with increased perinatal morbidity and mortality and usually warrant hospitalization for further evaluation or delivery.

The biophysical profile is a reliable predictor of fetal well-being. The false-negative rate is superior to that of the nonstress test alone and compares favorably with the false-negative rate of the contraction stress test. One study reported a false-negative rate of 0.6/1000 among 12,620 women tested weekly with the biophysical profile.[19] Another study reported significantly lower rates of cesarean delivery for fetal distress (3% vs. 22%), low 5-minute Apgar scores (1.6% and 3.2% vs. 12.5%), and meconium aspiration syndrome when the last biophysical profile before delivery was normal versus when it was abnormal.[13] Among 19,221 referred high-risk pregnancies, Manning and colleagues[18] reported a false-negative rate of 0.7/1000. The false-positive rate of the biophysical profile varies with the score of the last test prior to delivery, ranging from 0% if the last biophysical profile score before delivery was 0, to more than 40% if the last biophysical profile score was 6.

Advantages and Limitations

Advantages of the biophysical profile include excellent sensitivity, a weekly testing interval, a low false-negative rate, and improved detection of structural fetal anomalies. The primary *limitation* is the requirement for personnel trained in sonographic visualization of the fetus. Additionally, although the duration of ultrasound observation is less than 10 minutes in the majority of cases, the complete biophysical profile is more time-consuming than other noninvasive tests. However, when all ultrasound variables are normal, addition of the nonstress test does not appear to alter the discriminative accuracy of the test.

THE MODIFIED BIOPHYSICAL PROFILE

The modified biophysical profile (MBPP) combines the strengths of the nonstress test (ease of use, low cost) and the complete biophysical profile (improved sensitivity, low false-negative rate), while minimizing the requirement for additional training in sonographic visualization of the fetus. The test is performed once to twice weekly and utilizes the nonstress test as a short-term marker of fetal status and the amniotic fluid volume (i.e., amniotic fluid index) as a marker of longer-term placental function.

Interpretation and Management

Interpretation of the nonstress test incorporates assessment of reactivity, baseline rate, variability, and fetal heart rate decelerations. Late, prolonged, or significant variable decelerations, particularly in the setting of low-normal amniotic fluid volume (amniotic fluid index 5-10 cm), are considered abnormal.

The amniotic fluid index is calculated as the sum of the deepest vertical cord-free pockets of amniotic fluid in each of the four uterine quadrants. Normal amniotic fluid index is equal to or greater than 10 cm. Low-normal amniotic fluid index is between 5 and 10 cm. Low amniotic fluid index, or oligohydramnios, is 5 cm or less. The upper limit of normal amniotic fluid index (polyhydramnios) is in the range of 25 cm. Regardless of reactivity, oligohydramnios constitutes an abnormal test. If the modified biophysical profile is normal, the routine testing schedule is resumed.

If the modified biophysical profile is abnormal, a back-up test is warranted. The biophysical profile and the contraction stress test are the most common back-up tests and perform similarly with respect to perinatal morbidity and mortality. Further management is guided by the results of the back-up test. Management of the modified biophysical profile is summarized in Figure 9-2.

Nageotte and co-workers[30] evaluated 2774 high-risk pregnancies with twice-weekly modified biophysical profiles and reported one

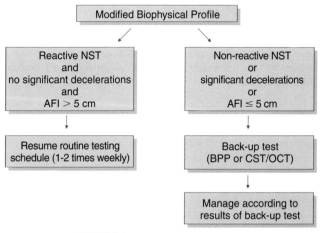

FIGURE 9-2 Management of the MBPP.

unexplained fetal death within 1 week of a normal test result, for a false-negative rate of 0.36/1000. Another study, by Miller and colleagues,[28] reported 54,617 modified biophysical profiles in 15,482 high-risk pregnancies. Antepartum testing in high-risk pregnancies yielded a fetal death rate that was nearly sevenfold lower than that in the untested, "low-risk" population. The overall false-negative rate of the modified biophysical profile was 0.8/1000, and the false-positive rate was 60%. Abnormal test results prompted intervention in 15.5% of the tested population; however, iatrogenic prematurity occurred in only 1.5% of women tested before 37 weeks. When the modified biophysical profile is used as described by Miller and Nageotte, the amniotic fluid index is repeated twice weekly. Alternatively, weekly amniotic fluid index determinations may be reasonable prior to 41 weeks, provided that the amniotic fluid index remains greater than 8 cm.[16,41] Beyond 41 weeks, oligohydramnios may develop more rapidly, and the amniotic fluid index should be assessed twice weekly. Large studies reveal the false-negative rate of the modified biophysical profile to be similar to that of the contraction stress test and the complete biophysical profile.

Advantages and Limitations

Advantages of the modified biophysical profile are that it is easier to perform and less time-consuming than the contraction stress test or

the complete biophysical profile. The sensitivity of the modified biophysical profile is superior to that of the nonstress test alone. *Limitations* include the need for back-up testing in 10% to 50% of patients,
a high false-positive rate, and a twice-weekly testing interval.
Figure 9-2 depicts a schematic for management of the modified
biophysical profile.

FETAL MOVEMENT COUNTS

Maternal perception of normal fetal movement has long been recognized as a reliable indicator of fetal well-being. Conversely, prolonged absence of fetal movement may signal fetal death. Whereas
cessation of fetal movement in response to hypoxia has been demonstrated in animal studies, controlled data in human fetuses are lacking. Nevertheless, any acute decrement in the number or strength of
fetal movements should raise the suspicion of fetal compromise and
should prompt further evaluation. Many clinicians recommend routine fetal movement counting, particularly in women who are considered high risk.[11,29,33]

Interpretation and Management

A common approach is to recommend the pregnant woman count
fetal movements for 1 hour each day.

- Ten fetal movements in a 1-hour period are considered
  reassuring.
- If fewer than ten movements are perceived, counting is
  continued for another hour.
- Fewer than ten movements in a 2-hour period should alert the
  patient to contact her physician for further evaluation.

Another approach calls for the pregnant woman to count movements
for 1 hour three times per week. A third protocol calls for movement
counting two to three times daily for 30 minutes. With this latter
approach, further evaluation is recommended if there are fewer than
four strong movements in a 30-minute period.

Evidence from one study using non-concurrent controls demonstrated a lower rate of fetal death and a higher incidence of intervention for fetal distress in patients using a formalized protocol of fetal
movement counting.[29] Fetal movement counting is an inexpensive
method of involving the patient in her own care and may be a valuable adjunct to routine prenatal care, regardless of risk category.

UMBILICAL ARTERY DOPPLER VELOCIMETRY

Doppler velocimetry of fetal, umbilical, and uterine vessels has been the focus of intensive study in recent years. This technology utilizes systolic/diastolic flow ratios and resistance indices to estimate blood flow in various arteries. Recent studies have shown statistically significant improvement in perinatal outcome with the use of Doppler ultrasonography in pregnancies complicated by fetal growth restriction.[1,26] Although severe restriction of umbilical artery blood flow—as evidenced by absent or reversed flow during diastole—has been correlated with fetal growth restriction, acidosis, and adverse perinatal outcome, the predictive values of less extreme deviations from normal remain undefined. In conditions other than fetal growth restriction, Doppler velocimetry does not appear to be a useful screening test for the detection of fetal compromise, and it is not recommended for use as a screening test in the general obstetric population.

Doppler velocimetry of the middle cerebral artery demonstrates increased diastolic flow in the setting of reduced fetal oxygenation, reflecting the "brain-sparing" effect of hypoxemia.[3] The peak systolic velocity in the middle cerebral artery has been shown to increase significantly in the setting of fetal anemia and can predict moderate to severe anemia with sensitivity and negative predictive values that equal or exceed those of the traditional method of amniocentesis for Δ OD 450 determination.[7,21-25]

A number of studies have evaluated the utility of uterine artery Doppler waveform analysis in the prediction of fetal growth restriction.[34] In the setting of an abnormal uterine artery Doppler waveform, the pooled likelihood ratio was 3.67. When Doppler velocimetry measurements are used in antepartum fetal surveillance, they should be interpreted in the context of the clinical setting and the results of other tests of fetal status.

BIOCHEMICAL ASSESSMENT

Amniocentesis for Fetal Lung Maturity

Amniocentesis is an invasive procedure in which a needle is introduced into the amniotic cavity to remove amniotic fluid for analysis. It is performed under ultrasound guidance using a 20- to 22-gauge spinal-type needle placed transabdominally to withdraw 5 to 20 ml

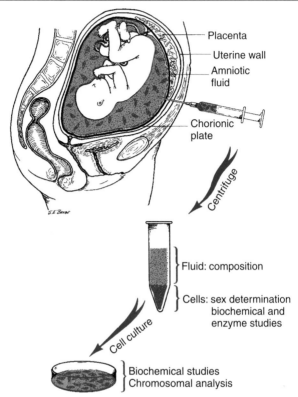

FIGURE 9-3 Amniocentesis. Amniotic fluid is aspirated with a sterile syringe. The sample is centrifuged to separate cells and fluid.

of amniotic fluid (Figure 9-3). In the second trimester, amniocentesis is used frequently to detect a number of abnormalities, including aneuploidy. In the third trimester, it is used primarily to assess fetal lung maturity. Risks in the third trimester are relatively few and include bleeding, infection, membrane rupture, preterm labor, preterm delivery, and possibly alloimmunization in the setting of blood type incompatibility. Amniotic fluid can be used to assess fetal lung maturity by a number of methods.

Lecithin-to-Sphingomyelin Ratio

Pulmonary surfactant contains primarily phospholipids. Surfactant acts as a surface detergent at the air–liquid interface of the alveoli, preventing collapse at the end of expiration. The lecithin-to-sphingomyelin (L/S) ratio compares the concentrations of two phospholipids, lecithin and sphingomyelin, that are major components of surfactant. In the third trimester, an increase in lecithin causes a rise in the lecithin-to-sphingomyelin ratio. A ratio of 2.0 or greater is associated with a low risk of neonatal surfactant-deficient respiratory distress syndrome (RDS).

The following interpretation is generally accepted:

L/S Ratio	Fetal Lung	Risk for RDS
>2.0	Mature	Minimal
1.5–2.0	Transitional	Moderate
<1.5	Immature	High

Note that the presence of blood or meconium can interfere with the results of the lecithin-to-sphingomyelin ratio.

Foam Stability Test

This test is based on the ability of surfactant to generate stable foam when ethanol is added to the amniotic fluid specimen. Ethanol, isotonic saline, and amniotic fluid at varying dilutions are shaken together for 15 seconds. At the proper dilution, a ring of bubbles at the air–liquid interface after 15 minutes indicates probable fetal lung maturity (Figure 9-4).

Phosphatidylglycerol

The presence of phosphatidylglycerol can be ascertained quickly and is not impacted by blood or meconium. The presence of phosphatidylglycerol indicates a low risk for respiratory distress

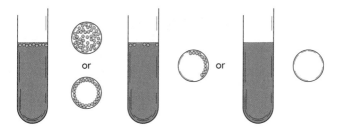

Positive foam test   Negative foam test

FIGURE 9-4 Foam stability test (shake test). For the test to be positive, bubbles must be seen around the entire circumference of tube.

syndrome. Whenever possible, fetal lung maturity assessment should be based on phosphatidylglycerol in combination with the lecithin-to-sphingomyelin ratio.

Fluorescence Polarization (FLM-II Assay)

The fetal lung maturity (FLM-II) assay uses fluorescence polarization to determine lipid membrane fluidity in amniotic fluid.

Interpretation of the FLM-II assay is summarized below:

Mature	>55 mg/g
Transitional	40–54 mg/g
Immature	<39 mg/g

Lamellar Body Count

Lamellar body counting measures the number of surfactant-containing particles in amniotic fluid directly by using the platelet channel of a standard hematology cell counter. The size and number of lamellar bodies in the amniotic fluid are predictive of fetal lung maturity.[32] Interpretation is summarized below:

Mature	$\geq$50,000/μL
Transitional	>15,000 to <50,000/μL
Immature	$\leq$15,000/μL

SUMMARY

Our ability to assess the condition of the fetus has improved dramatically over the past 40 years. Although diagnostic precision is enhanced by electronic fetal heart rate monitoring and ultrasound technology, room for improvement remains. Electronic fetal heart rate monitoring is a very sensitive tool for the detection of disrupted fetal oxygenation; truly compromised fetuses rarely fail to exhibit abnormal fetal heart rate patterns. The converse, however, is not true. Fetal heart rate patterns such as decelerations, tachycardia, and intermittent reduction in variability and/or accelerations frequently are observed in the absence of fetal compromise. The limited positive predictive value is the principle shortcoming of fetal heart rate monitoring. Accuracy may be improved by combining fetal heart rate analysis with assessment of biophysical variables, such as amniotic fluid volume, fetal movement, breathing, tone, and blood flow characteristics. To date, the most effective combination of variables has not been defined, and no one approach to fetal surveillance has demonstrated clear superiority over the others. Yet, despite the limitations, antepartum testing in high-risk pregnancies has been reported to yield a fetal death rate lower than that observed in untested, low-risk pregnancies.[28] If this observation is substantiated, future investigation will be needed to address the role of antepartum fetal surveillance in uncomplicated, low-risk pregnancies.

References

1. Alfirevic Z, Neilson JP: Doppler ultrasonography in high-risk pregnancies: Systematic review with meta-analysis, *Am J Obstet Gynecol* 172 (5):1379-1387, 1995.

2. American College of Obstetricians and Gynecologists: Intrapartum fetal heart rate monitoring, ACOG *Practice Bulletin* no.70, *Obstet Gynecol* 106(6):1453-1461, 2005.

3. Bahado-Singh RO, Kovanci E, Jeffres A, Oz U, Deren O, Copel J, Mari G: The Doppler cerebroplacental ratio and perinatal outcome in intrauterine growth restriction, *Am J Obstet Gynecol* 180(3 Pt 1):750-756, 1999.

4. Boehm FH, Salyer S, Shah DM, Vaughn WK: Improved outcome of twice weekly nonstress testing, *Obstet Gynecol* 67(4):566-568, 1986.

5. Clark SL, Gimovsky ML, Miller FC: The scalp stimulation test: A clinical alternative to fetal scalp blood sampling, *Am J Obstet Gynecol* 148 (3):274-277, 1984.

6. Clark SL, Gimovsky ML, Miller FC: Fetal heart rate response to scalp blood sampling, *Am J Obstet Gynecol* 144(6):706-708, 1982.

7. Dukler D, Oepkes D, Seaward G, Windrim R, Ryan G: Noninvasive tests to predict fetal anemia: A study comparing Doppler and ultrasound parameters, *Am J Obstet Gynecol* 188(5):1310-1314, 2003.

8. Edersheim TG, Hutson JM, Druzin ML, Kogut EA: Fetal heart rate response to vibratory acoustic stimulation predicts fetal pH in labor, *Am J Obstet Gynecol* 157(6):1557-1560, 1987.

9. Elimian A, Figueroa R, Tejani N: Intrapartum assessment of fetal well-being: A comparison of scalp stimulation with scalp blood pH sampling, *Obstet Gynecol* 89(3):373-376, 1987.

10. Freeman RK, Anderson G, Dorchester W: A prospective multi-institutional study of antepartum fetal heart rate monitoring. II. Contraction stress test versus nonstress test for primary surveillance, *Am J Obstet Gynecol* 143(7):778-781, 1982.

11. Grant A, Elbourne D, Valentin L, Alexander S: Routine formal fetal movement counting and risk of antepartum late death in normally formed singletons, *Lancet* 2(8659):345-349, 1989.

12. Ingemarsson I, Arulkumaran S: Reactive fetal heart rate response to VAS in fetuses with low scalp blood pH, *Br J Obstet Gynaecol* 96(5):562-565, 1989.

13. Johnson JM, Harman CR, Lange IR, Manning FA: Biophysical profile scoring in the management of postterm pregnancy: an analysis of 307 patients, *Am J Obstet Gynecol* 154(2):269-273, 1986.

14. Kubli FW, Hon EH, Khazin AF, Takemura H: Observations on heart rate and pH in the human fetus during labor, *Am J Obstet Gynecol* 104(8): 1190-1206, 1969.

15. Lagrew DC Jr: The contraction stress test, *Clin Obstet Gynecol* 38(1): 11-25, 1995.

16. Lagrew DC, Pircon RA, Nageotte M, Freeman RK, Dorchester W: How frequently should the amniotic fluid index be repeated? *Am J Obstet Gynecol* 167(4 Pt 1):1129-1133, 1992.

17. Manning FA, Lange IR, Morrison I, Harman CR: Determination of fetal health: Methods for antepartum and intrapartum fetal assessment, *Curr Prob Obstet Gynecol* 7:3, 1983.

18. Manning FA, Morrison I, Harman CR, Lange IR, Menticoglou S: Fetal assessment based on fetal biophysical profile scoring: experience in 19,221 referred high-risk pregnancies. II. An analysis of false-negative fetal deaths, *Am J Obstet Gynecol* 157(4 Pt 1):880-884, 1987.

19. Manning FA, Morrison I, Lange IR, Harman CR, Chamberlain PF: Fetal assessment based upon fetal BPP scoring: Experience in 12,620 referred high risk pregnancies. I. Perinatal mortality by frequency and etiology, *Am J Obstet Gynecol* 151(3):343-350, 1985.

20. Manning FA, Platt LD, Sipos L: Antepartum fetal evaluation: Development of a fetal biophysical profile, *Am J Obstet Gynecol* 136(6): 787-795, 1980.

21. Mari G, Adrignolo A, Abuhamad AZ, Pirhonen J, Jones DC, Ludomirsky A, Copel JA: Diagnosis of fetal anemia with Doppler ultrasound in the pregnancy complicated by maternal blood group immunization, *Ultrasound Obstet Gynecol* 5(6):400-405, 1995.

22. Mari G, Deter RL, Carpenter RL, Rahman F, Zimmerman R, Moise KJ Jr, Dorman KF, Ludomirsky A, Gonzalez R, Gomez R, Oz U, Detti L, Copel JA, Bahado-Singh R, Berry S, Martinez-Poyer J, Blackwell SC: Noninvasive diagnosis by Doppler ultrasonography of fetal anemia due to maternal red cell alloimmunization, Collaborative Group for Doppler Assessment of the Blood Velocity in Anemic Fetuses, *N Engl J Med* 342 (1):9-14, 2000.

23. Mari G, Detti L, Oz U, Zimmerman R, Duerig P, Stefos T: Accurate prediction of fetal hemoglobin by Doppler ultrasonography, *Obstet Gynecol* 99(4):589-593, 2002.

24. Mari G, Hanif F, Kruger M, Cosmi E, Santolaya-Forgas J, Treadwell MC: Middle cerebral artery peak systolic velocity: A new Doppler parameter in the assessment of growth-restricted fetuses, *Ultrasound Obstet Gynecol* 29(3):310-316, 2007.

25. Mari G, Rahman F, Olofsson P, Ozcan T, Copel JA: Increase of fetal hematocrit decreases the middle cerebral artery peak systolic velocity in pregnancies complicated by rhesus alloimmunization, *J Matern Fetal Med* 6(4):206-208, 1997.

26. Maulik D: Doppler ultrasound in obstetrics. In Cunningham G, MacDonald P, Gant N, Leveno K, Gilstrap L, editors: *Williams obstetrics supplement*, Stanford, CT, 1996, Appleton and Lange.

27. Meis PJ, Ureda JR, Swain M, Kelly RT, Penry M, Sharp P: Variable decelerations during nonstress tests are not a sign of fetal compromise, *Am J Obstet Gynecol* 154(3):586-590, 1986.

28. Miller DA, Rabello YA, Paul RH: The modified biophysical profile: antepartum testing in the 1990s, *Am J Obstet Gynecol* 174(3):812-817, 1996.

29. Moore TR, Piacquadio K: A prospective evaluation of fetal movement screening to reduce the incidence of antepartum fetal death, *Am J Obstet Gynecol* 60(5 Pt 1):1075-1080, 1989.

30. Nageotte JP, Towers CV, Asrat T, Freeman RK: Perinatal outcome with the MBPP, *Am J Obstet Gynecol* 170(6):1672-1676, 1994.

31. National Institute of Child Health and Human Development Research Planning Workshop: Electronic fetal heart rate monitoring: Research guidelines for interpretation, *Am J Obstet Gynecol* 177(6):1385-1390, 1997.

32. Neerhof MG, Dohnal JC, Ashwood ER, Lee IS, Anceschi MM: Lamellar body counts: A consensus on protocol, *Obstet Gynecol* 97(2):318-320, 2001.

33. Neldam S: Fetal movements as an indicator of fetal well-being, *Dan Med Bull* 30(4):274-278, 1983.

34. Papageorghiou AT, Yu CK, Nicolaides KH: The role of uterine artery Doppler in predicting adverse pregnancy outcome, *Best Pract Res Clin Obstet Gynaecol* 18(3):383-396, 2004.

35. Phelan JP, Lewis PE Jr: Fetal heart rate decelerations during a nonstress test, *Obstet Gynecol* 57(2):228-232, 1981.

36. Phelan JP, Platt LD, Yeh SY, Trujillo M, Paul RH: Continuing role of the non-stress test in the management of post-dates pregnancy, *Obstet Gynecol* 64(5):624-628, 1984.

37. Polzin GB, Blakemore KJ, Petrie RH, Amon E: Fetal vibro-acoustic stimulation: Magnitude and duration of fetal heart rate accelerations as a marker of fetal health, *Obstet Gynecol* 72(4):621-626, 1988.

38. Skupski DW, Rosenberg CR, Eglington GS: Intrapartum fetal stimulation tests: A meta-analysis, *Obstet Gynecol* 99(1):129-134, 2002.

39. Smith CV, Nguyen HN, Phelan JP, Paul RH: Intrapartum assessment of fetal well-being: A comparison of fetal acoustic stimulation with acid-base determinations, *Am J Obstet Gynecol* 155(4):726-728, 1986.

40. Spencer JA: Predictive value of a fetal heart rate acceleration at the time of fetal blood sampling in labour, *J Perinat Med* 19(3):207-215, 1991.

41. Wing DA, Fishman A, Gonzalez C, Paul RH: How frequently should the amniotic fluid index be performed during the course of antepartum testing? *Am J Obstet Gynecol* 174(1 Pt 1):33-36, 1996.

CHAPTER 10

Patient Safety, Risk Management, and Documentation

K ey components of a successful risk management program are avoiding preventable adverse outcomes and decreasing the risk of liability exposure.[53] Liability exposure is nonexistent without perinatal morbidity, mortality, or both. Several studies suggest that significant decreases in perinatal morbidity and mortality related to intrapartum asphyxia, low Apgar scores, hypoxic-ischemic encephalopathy, and suboptimal obstetric care are attainable goals for perinatal services. A patient safety approach to perinatal care is the key to meeting these goals and has been successfully implemented in a variety of institutions both in the United States and abroad.[9,11,31,60] The focus of this chapter is to provide some understanding of human error, to identify sources of potential errors related to perinatal care and electronic fetal monitoring (EFM), to suggest strategies that may prevent or reduce errors, and to review approaches to assessment, communication, and documentation that promote optimal outcomes. Additionally, documentation issues specific to electronic fetal monitoring and related medical-legal concerns are addressed.

OCCURRENCE OF ERRORS

Errors occur in every industry, and the occurrence of errors in health care is nothing new. The report, *To Err Is Human: Building a Safer Health System*, published by the Institute of Medicine[19] from its Committee on Quality of Health Care in America, brought national attention to statistics identifying medical errors as a significant cause of patient death or injury. Typical errors in health care settings relate to misunderstandings, erroneous use of medical devices, medication errors, lack of communication as patients move from one setting or one care provider to the next, unintended acts of omission such as not doing or responding to something, and acts of commission such as doing something outside the standard of care or practice. The Institute of Medicine report[19] advocated a shift, when patient injuries occur, from the old paradigm of "blame and train" to identifying underlying system failures that have contributed to the preventable adverse outcome.

Through the efforts of the Joint Commission for the Accreditation of Healthcare Organizations (The Joint Commission), the Agency for Healthcare Research and Quality, and other organizations engaged in quality improvement in health care, patient safety has been established as the first priority in health care. The analysis of large numbers of injuries and reported errors confirms that adverse events most often result from error-prone systems and processes, not from error-prone individuals. Organizations must learn to avoid the "conspiracy of silence" and create systems where errors can be identified and prevention strategies can be developed.[10]

Human Error

Health care providers are educated and socialized to "do the right thing"—that is, to provide safe and appropriate care that results in a positive outcome. However, all health care providers are human, and humans make errors. Error is a normal part of the human experience and does not reflect laziness, bad intentions, or a personality defect.[43] Understanding the nature of human errors (human factor analysis) is essential to any effort to prevent them. The *most common types of human error are related to slips, trips, and lapses*,[43] which occur throughout a wide range of human activity. The following lists these activities in decreasing order of probability of occurrence:[40,50]

- Stress (lack of time combined with high stakes—e.g., wrong sponge count in crash surgery)
- Change of shift (e.g., miscommunication)
- Inspection or monitoring (e.g., missing or not recognizing something)
- Arithmetic (e.g., miscalculating drug dosage)
- Omission (e.g., not doing or responding appropriately to something)
- Commission (doing something that is not consistent with an accepted standard of care)

Human errors *are more likely to occur in the presence of personal and environmental factors* known to increase the risk of error. Specific conditions have been identified that are known to increase the risk of error, and it is helpful to be aware of them. These conditions, listed in decreasing probability of risk of error, include the following:[43,50,59]

1. Lack of familiarity with a task
2. Shortage of time
3. Poor communication
4. Information overload
5. Misperception of risk
6. Lack of experience (not necessarily training)
7. Poor instructions or procedures
8. Inadequate checking
9. Educational mismatch of a person with the task
10. Disturbed sleep pattern
11. Hostile environment
12. Monotony and boredom

Being aware of the most common types of errors and error-producing conditions helps in identifying, reducing, and managing risks in the perinatal setting. It is also helpful to understand human performance as it relates to knowledge, application of rules, and skills. For example, nurses function from a specialized knowledge base. As they become more skilled and experienced, they process information rapidly in recurrent activities and perform many duties automatically.[42] *Skill-based performance* includes starting a routine intravenous line, applying the external fetal monitor, and performing Leopold's maneuvers. Errors can occur when nurses' routines change or their attention is diverted, or from physiologic (fatigue, illness), psychologic (stress, family issues, frustration), or environmental (noise or unusual unit activity) factors.

Rule-based performance requires extra attention when an event differs from the routine. For example, when confronted with a commonly occurring problem, such as onset of fetal heart rate (FHR) variable decelerations, experienced nurses operate from known and practiced rules or a series of learned responses for doing X when Y happens. When an unfamiliar problem arises, a rule-based error may occur because the wrong rule is chosen, the situation is not accurately perceived, or the rule is misapplied.[42]

Knowledge-based performance requires controlled and conscious thought when nurses encounter a completely new, unfamiliar, or infrequently occurring situation. Examples of this type of situation are acute uterine rupture, development of a rarely seen sinusoidal fetal heart rate pattern, unheralded prolonged fetal heart rate deceleration to 60 beats per minute or less, or maternal seizure in the absence of a known seizure-related condition. Errors can occur because of lack of information or data, or from misdirected attempts to match this novel situation to previous and more familiar situations. As the expertise of the nurse increases, the focus of control moves from a knowledge-based and rule-based performance to skill-based functions. What was once novel has become routine and the nurse does not usually have to resort to knowledge-based reasoning.[42]

In summary, not all errors are preventable. And although humans do err, errors do not always result in injury or adverse outcomes, and not all adverse outcomes are the result of error.[42] It is unreasonable to presume that any one individual is the only person responsible for an error that results in injury to a patient. *It is inappropriate to rely on prevention of error as the sole means of creating patient safety.* Systems should be in place that will catch errors before they result in adverse outcomes; however, systems are subject to human and environmental variations. The role of risk management in the perinatal setting is twofold: (1) to reduce the probability that a given risk will result in a poor outcome, and (2) to recognize, mitigate, or minimize the consequences of the event rather than relying on prevention of error as the sole means of creating patient safety.[47,53]

Common Errors in Perinatal Care

The most common errors leading to injury in perinatal care are as follows:*

- Lack of accurate interpretation of fetal monitoring, resulting in lack of timely recognition of both antepartum and intrapartum fetal compromise
- Lack of appropriate response to nonreassuring FHR tracings
- Delay in decision for, or initiation of, cesarean or operative vaginal delivery as indicated by fetal or maternal status
- Lack of appropriate skills to perform neonatal resuscitation
- Non-indicated use of induction or augmentation of labor; failure to discontinue uterine stimulants in the presence of nonreassuring FHR pattern; excessive dosages of uterine stimulants resulting in hyperactivity or uterine rupture
- Inappropriate use of forceps or vacuum extractor resulting in fetal trauma
- Application of fundal pressure
- Lack of communication between care providers (not done, not clear, not documented)
- Incomplete documentation

---

*References 22,26,47,50,51,53

Electronic fetal monitoring continues to be an area that has great potential for error, in part due to the wide variance in electronic fetal monitoring education both between and among the disciplines of nursing, midwifery, and medicine.[36] Electronic fetal monitoring interpretation issues have been linked to avoidable intrapartum fetal demise and "[have] become the dominant litigation theme internationally."[60] Clinicians are best served by advancing approaches to electronic fetal monitoring interpretation and management that are based on patient safety principles, such as the development of high-reliability perinatal units.

PREVENTION OF ERRORS AND RISK REDUCTION

High-Reliability Perinatal Units

Risk reduction and error prevention in perinatal care can be achieved when organizations direct their efforts to the avoidance of these common situations and foster high-reliability characteristics. *High reliability* is defined as the technical ability to operate technologically complex systems essentially without error over long periods of time. There are organizational characteristics and clinical practices that differentiate highly reliable perinatal units from those experiencing more error and injury. These organizations consider patient safety to be the first priority and have systems in place to prevent recognized sources of error and injury. The primary characteristics of a high-reliability unit are as follows:[25,26,37,45,46]

- The organization creates and fosters a safety-oriented culture.
- Decision making to enhance safety occurs at every level of the organization.
- Alarms can be called by anyone; hierarchy is minimized, rank is not an issue; anyone can challenge the status quo.
- Jobs are designed for safety; there is minimal reliance on memory; protocols, checklists, and forcing functions are built into the system.
- Teams that are expected to work together (e.g., physicians, midwives, and nurses participating in the same advanced fetal monitoring workshops) are trained and educated together.
- Multidisciplinary teams carry out drills for high-risk situations such as emergency cesarean deliveries.
- Communication is continuous, valued, and highly rewarded.

- The organization promotes the development of competencies and evaluates ongoing competence using a variety of learning techniques such as simulations, computer tutorials, and case studies in fetal monitoring.

There are many tools and resources for promoting high reliability in perinatal care, and hospitals should explore a variety of methods to reach these goals. One approach to the development of high-reliability perinatal care is to consistently promote patient care within a model such as the Circle of Safety™.

Creating a Circle of Safety™

A concept developed to promote a systematic approach to patient safety in perinatal care is the Circle of Safety™. It consists of three main components: *Clinical Comprehension, Communication, & Collaboration* (Figure 10-1). Note that these three components are inextricably linked and all must be present to achieve patient safety.

- ***Clinical Comprehension*** encompasses the knowledge base of the involved clinicians based on their training, education, and expertise in conjunction with specific individual patient information, such as risk factors and clinical context. It forms the foundation for safe patient care. If clinical comprehension is

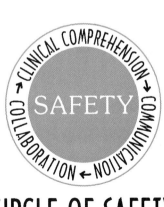

CIRCLE OF SAFETY™

FIGURE 10-1 Schematic representation of the three elements of practice comprising the Circle of Safety™ approach: Clinical Comprehension, Communication, & Collaboration. (Courtesy Perinatal Risk Management & Education Services, Chicago, IL.)

missing, both communication and collaboration will be adversely affected.

- *Communication* refers to the ongoing dialogue between team members, including the patient and family members. Communication among clinicians may be based on a guide such as SBAR (situation, background, assessment, recommendation[17,28]) or the 5-step assertiveness[35] script. Communication also includes discussions with the patient and family, such as informed consent, informed refusal, and disclosure. Appropriate communication is based on clinical knowledge and comprehension, which are the keys to effective collaboration. Samples of communication using SBAR and 5-step assertiveness in the perinatal setting are provided in Box 10-1 and Box 10-2.

BOX 10-1   Sample Communication Related to Electronic Fetal Monitoring Using SBAR

1. **Situation:** State what is happening at the present time; state the circumstances that prompted the communication.
   "Hi Dr. Johnson, it's Sue from L & D. Mrs. Smith, your patient in active labor who requested an epidural, is having a FHR pattern that is confusing to me. I can't tell if the changes are accelerations or decelerations."
2. **Background:** Put the situation into context; explain any pertinent background information.
   "She's a G2P1001, her last exam was 30 minutes ago, and she was 5 cm/100%/Vtx 1 with SROM clear since 0930. She has no noted risk factors."
3. **Assessment:** Explain what you think the problem is; include pertinent assessments.
   "I'm not sure the external monitor is picking up well. The prior baseline was 140 with moderate variability and no accels or decels. Now it's hard to tell, but I think the baseline has risen to 150, but it may have dropped to 130, there's minimal variability, and depending on where I read the baseline we have either accels or decels."
4. **Recommendation:** Express your thoughts on a solution. Be direct in asking for what you want to see happen.
   "If it's OK with you I'd like to hold off on the epidural placement until I can get a clear reading on this tracing. I've paged the resident to come look at it with me, and if we can't figure it out I may ask you to come to the bedside for an evaluation."

Adapted from Leonard M, Graham S, Bonacrum D: The human factor: The critical importance of effective teamwork and communication in providing safe care, *Qual Saf Health* 13(suppl 1):i85-i90, 2004, and Haig KM, Sutton S, Whittington J: SBAR: A shared mental model for improving communication between clinicians, *Jt Comm J Qual Patient Saf* 32(3):167-175, 2006.

BOX 10-2   Sample Communication Related to Electronic Fetal Monitoring Using 5-Step Assertiveness

1. **Use a name or position to get the team member's attention.**
   "Dr. Johnson."
2. **Express your discomfort.**
   "Dr. Johnson, I'm uncomfortable with proceeding with the epidural."
3. **Clearly and candidly state your concern.**
   "Dr. Johnson, I'm uncomfortable with proceeding with the epidural because I can't determine whether these are accels or decels."
4. **Propose an alternative.**
   "Dr. Johnson, I'm uncomfortable with proceeding with the epidural because I can't determine whether these are accels or decels. I'd like to adjust the monitor and have you come evaluate the tracing with me before we proceed with the epidural."
5. **Obtain acknowledgment.**
   "Dr. Johnson, I'm uncomfortable with proceeding with the epidural because I can't determine whether these are accels or decels. I'd like to adjust the monitor and have you come evaluate the tracing with me before we proceed with the epidural. OK with you?"

Adapted from Miller LA: Patient safety and teamwork in perinatal care, *J Perinat Neonatal Nurs* 19(1):46-51, 2005.

Hospital cultures that promote respectful conflict resolution and encourage direct communication experience improved nursing job satisfaction and a subsequent positive impact on both patient safety and evidence-based perinatal care.[57]

- *Collaboration* occurs when clinicians form a plan of care that supports the patient and family and incorporates evidence-based practices and ongoing evaluation. Collaboration is a key process in achieving safety, often leading to new clinical comprehension regarding patient care and thus bringing the clinicians "full circle" in a safety-based approach.

A case management illustration using the principles of clinical comprehension, communication, and collaboration outlined above can be found in Figure 10-2. In this case, a 24-year-old Gravida 2, Para 1 with a normal prenatal course and no risk factors had been ambulating in active labor following a normal electronic fetal monitoring tracing (Figure 10-2A). She was being followed by a certified nurse-midwife (CNM) who was on the labor and delivery unit. Returning to the room for reapplication of electronic fetal monitoring, the registered nurse (RN) had difficulty obtaining the fetal heart rate. This was noted on the central monitor by another registered nurse, who notified the certified nurse-midwife, and both

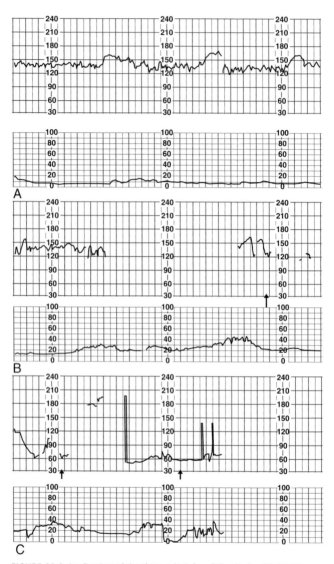

FIGURE 10-2 Application of the three principles of the Circle of Safety™ approach. **A.** FHR tracing prior to ambulation, all components normal. **B.** RN at desk notes irregularity on central display (*arrow*), notifies CNM, and both respond by going to labor room. **C.** *First arrow*: FHR audibly noted below normal, artificial rupture of membranes reveals bloody fluid, FSE placed and intrauterine resuscitation is begun. *Second arrow*: CNM decision to move patient to operating suite, team notified to assemble there. (Courtesy Perinatal Risk Management & Education Services, Chicago, IL.)

went immediately to the labor room to assess and offer assistance (Figure 10-2B). A fetal heart rate below normal was audible, and the certified nurse-midwife performed a vaginal exam, artificially ruptured membranes (revealing approximately 2 cups of bright red bloody fluid), and applied a fetal scalp electrode.

Bradycardia was noted and intrauterine resuscitation was begun (Figure 10-2C). The certified nurse-midwife called for the patient to be prepped and moved to the operating suite for probable cesarean delivery. She also asked for notification of the physician and other support staff, including the pediatric/neonatal resuscitation team. Throughout the process the patient and family were apprised of the situation and given clear instructions and information as to the plan of action. The physician met the team in the operating suite and was given a quick report by the certified nurse-midwife. At this juncture, it was noted that although anesthesia had been paged and had responded, they had not yet arrived. The fetal heart rate remained bradycardic with absent variability, and the frank vaginal bleeding had continued. A second page to anesthesia was requested, and the certified nurse-midwife suggested use of local anesthesia should the anesthesiologist not arrive within the next 30 seconds. The physician agreed, but anesthesia arrived prior to the time limit and the patient was given general anesthesia. The infant was delivered and resuscitated successfully, resulting in Apgar scores of 6 and 9. Cord gases revealed metabolic acidosis in the umbilical artery, with only a respiratory acidosis in the umbilical vein, findings consistent with a short duration insult. Placental examination revealed an abruption of approximately 40%, confirmed by pathology studies. The time from the certified nurse-midwife deciding to move the patient to the operating suite to the actual delivery of the infant was *nine minutes*.

This case exemplifies the Circle of Safety™ methodology. The team (registered nurses and certified nurse-midwife) had the requisite *clinical comprehension;* that is, they recognized what was likely an abruption and the seriousness of fetal heart rate findings in context. *Communication* was direct and clear, with each team member understanding his or her role and responding quickly and professionally. Team *collaboration* was evident throughout the case, from the initial response of the registered nurse at the central display to the communication between the certified nurse-midwife and physician in the operating suite. Prior to this event, the hospital had completed multidisciplinary education in the areas of electronic fetal monitoring, emergency response, and teamwork and had a policy in place that encouraged nurses and certified nurse-midwives to anticipate the need for emergent delivery and move the patient without waiting for a physician to arrive at the bedside. Physicians had been trained to respond immediately and to meet the team in the operating suite where they could make the ultimate decision regarding delivery. This tactic allows significant delays to be avoided, while respecting the physician's ultimate decision on mode of delivery.

Following the application of an ongoing Circle of Safety™ approach to a specific situation encourages clinicians to constantly review and reformulate management plans in light of a changing clinical context. It recognizes the importance of a team approach, with clear communication among clinicians, as well as among patients, family members, and clinicians, and underscores the importance of creating a well-defined plan and re-evaluating the plan as labor progresses. When the plan is followed with regard to fetal heart rate tracing evaluation, it fits seamlessly with the standardized management decision model presented in Chapter 6.

Guidelines to Promote Safety and Reduce Risks

Recommendations and guidelines to promote patient safety and to decrease risk exposure include the following:[7,21,47,53]

Policies, Procedures, and Protocols

- Develop policies, procedures, and protocols based on accepted standards of care.[15,27,34]
- Create departmental policies (vs. nursing policies) for areas of practice that are interdisciplinary by nature (EFM, labor induction/augmentation) and attempt to standardize care whenever possible.
- Use guidelines promulgated by professional organizations (e.g., Association of Women's Health, Obstetric and Neonatal Nurses, American College of Obstetricians and Gynecologists, Society of Gynecologists and Obstetricians of Canada), journals, textbooks, and particularly evidence-based practice reports as sources for developing policies, procedures, and protocols.[30]

Competency

- Verify nurses' qualifications at the time of hire to ensure that they meet the prerequisites of the institution.
- Develop tools to evaluate performance related to specific skills, knowledge base of physiology and pathophysiology, and the

standard of care to which nurses are held accountable, based on the facility's rules (i.e., policies, procedures, and protocols).[34]

- Promote and support certification of nurses in fetal monitoring.[44]
- Require midwives and physicians to hold certification in EFM as part of their credentialing process.

Fetal Monitoring

- Standardize fetal assessment and monitoring language throughout the institution, and clarify definitions for fetal well-being and assessment.[1,38]
- Accurately monitor FHR and uterine activity; use instrumentation appropriately.
- Identify and interpret EFM data accurately.[3,4,8,29]
- Implement intrauterine resuscitation techniques to ameliorate nonreassuring FHR tracings (e.g., maternal repositioning, increasing fluids, oxygen).[8]
- Communicate findings and efforts to correct FHR changes to physician or midwife in a clear and unambiguous manner using SBAR[17,28] or 5-step assertiveness.[35]
- Continue fetal assessment until birth, including monitoring until the abdominal preparation is begun on women who are having a cesarean delivery.[1]

Neonatal Resuscitation

- Ensure availability of appropriately trained and certified staff; redeploy staff as necessary to provide optimal care.
- Prepare appropriate equipment and medications prior to delivery.

Organizational Resources and Systems to Support Timely Interventions

- Have sufficient staff or be able to redeploy staff as needed. During the intrapartum period, the nurse-to-patient ratio should be 1:2 or 1:1, depending on the stage of labor and the complexity of the situation.[1,7] Staffing should be sufficient to begin a cesarean delivery within 30 minutes of a physician's decision to operate. A more expeditious delivery (<30 minutes) may be necessary in cases of abruptio placentae, prolapse of the umbilical cord, hemorrhage secondary to placenta previa, and uterine rupture.[1]
- Have systems in place that ensure a physician's timely response to the perinatal unit when needed and requested (e.g., in cases of a nonreassuring FHR pattern, uterine hyperstimulation with

oxytocin with fetal intolerance to labor, vaginal birth after cesarean delivery). A policy that exists in high-reliability perinatal units is that "a physician will come to the unit when requested by a nurse" (Box 10-3).[26]

Perinatal Teamwork: Collaboration and Communication

- Recognize multidisciplinary teams as the unifying principle that creates operational excellence and success. "In any situation requiring a real-time combination of multiple skills, experiences and judgment, *teams,* as opposed to individuals, create superior performance".[52,p.56]
- Engage in team building through a multidisciplinary clinical practice or performance improvement committee to come to consensus on both routine and problematic practices, to improve communication, to build trust and confidence in one another, and to achieve performance goals.[23,52]
- Work toward creating a culture in which everyone feels free to ask for help.[18,58]
- Initiate formal team training, such as MedTeams®, or Kaiser Permanente's Perinatal Patient Safety Project, which may prevent 40% or more malpractice-related events in labor and delivery.[18,33]
- Utilize a variety of methodologies to measure and assess patient safety.[48]

BOX 10-3   Elements of Promoting Safety and Reducing Risk

1. Utilization of policies, procedures, and protocols to standardize care
2. Ensure competency of all clinicians via certification in EFM
3. Standardized definitions for fetal assessment and monitoring with clear and unambiguous communication among clinicians
4. Neonatal resuscitation certified staff and appropriate equipment
5. Organizational resources, sufficient staff, and systems to support timely interventions by all clinicians
6. Perinatal teamwork with multidisciplinary collaboration and communication
7. Interdisciplinary focused case reviews, proactive approach to improving systems, and elimination of a blame-based environment
8. Chain of communication that supports quality and safe patient care to reduce risks and adverse outcomes
9. Conduct joint multidisciplinary education of the perinatal team

Interdisciplinary Case Reviews

- Eliminate a blame-based environment.
- Focus reviews on the *six most common allegations* of obstetric malpractice claims.[22,58] These are:
  1. Failure to recognize or respond to nonreassuring fetal status
  2. Failure to do a timely delivery
  3. Failure to conduct proper resuscitation
  4. Negligently causing vacuum or forceps injuries
  5. Failure to prevent and manage shoulder dystocia
  6. Improper use of oxytocin
- Use a proactive approach, such as "failure to rescue"[49] to review processes related to EFM management. This approach does not require a sentinel event to trigger a review and allows hospitals to develop best-practice strategies as well as evaluate "near misses."
- Engage several reviewers when reviewing and classifying adverse events.[12]

Chain of Communication

- Develop a chain of communication (Figure 10-3) with key medical, nursing, administrative, and risk-management leaders.
- Implement the chain of communication when team members disagree (e.g., about tracing interpretation or management of the patient) or when the clinicians fail to respond.[16]
- Report to the quality/performance improvement committee any incidence of provider behavior that does not support quality or safe patient care, that increases risk to the patient, or that could contribute to an adverse outcome. If retaliation or retribution occurs, it should be reported as well. "When people fail to engage in respectful interactions, things can get dangerous."[26]

Joint Nurse/Provider Education

- Make EFM education a multidisciplinary event and teach all clinicians the standard management decision model presented in Chapter 6.
- Provide consistency of information and expectations, hold forums on skills (e.g., an emergency cesarean delivery drill), on conducting patient conferences, and on any other activities that involve multidisciplinary team members.
- Incorporate training on communication and teamwork into residency education.[55]

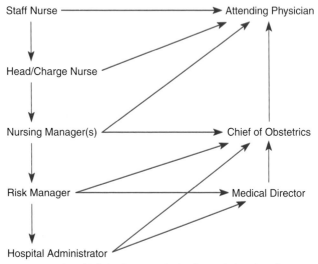

FIGURE 10-3 Sample chain of communication for resolution of conflicts in judgment between nurse and health care provider.

MANAGEMENT OF RISKS AND ADVERSE OUTCOMES

When there is litigation related to an adverse neonatal or maternal outcome, the physician, midwife, hospital, and, often, individual perinatal nurses are named as defendants.[54] Health care providers by nature and education want to help and care for people, so they are particularly devastated when they are sued by a client. The word *malpractice* evokes a guttural response in all health care providers, particularly in obstetrics where the damages are likely catastrophic with economic damages in the millions. Care providers fear being involved in malpractice suits and judged by a jury as liable in a situation where the care was, in fact, reasonable. They are likely to become preoccupied as unresolved lawsuits can take 3 or more years to be resolved.[41] But medical errors and litigation are a reality of practice. Acknowledging the risk and developing systems to reduce the risk and/or consequence of error is the first step in reducing medical-legal exposure. When risk issues or adverse outcomes are identified, the woman's medical record should be reviewed by the multidisciplinary health care team, utilizing an approach that will objectively analyze the clinical course to identify errors and contributing factors that may have resulted in an adverse outcome. Additionally, disclosure of adverse or unanticipated events to the patient and family is the responsibility of the health care team and may result in a reduction in legal action.[5] During the disclosure process, providers must maintain the patient relationship without compromising risk management.

Disclosure of Unanticipated Outcomes

When an injury occurs, The Joint Commission standards require that information about how the error occurred and remedies available be disclosed to the woman and her family.[20] During disclosure, the woman and her family should be informed that the factors involved in the injury will be investigated so that steps can be taken to reduce the likelihood of similar injury to other patients.[39] Disclosure should be made with the support of trained individuals; clinicians should refrain from discussing the details of the event with the patient and family without appropriate support through the organization's disclosure process. Institutions should provide education related to the components of disclosure, and several organizations have developed disclosure programs that can serve as models for disclosure in the perinatal setting.[14]

Elements of Malpractice

Failure to do something that a reasonable and prudent clinician would do in the same circumstances is known as malpractice or professional negligence. Clinicians are held to national standards of care and practice within the "same or similar circumstances" and "reasonably expected" parameters. Inherent in this statement is the expectation that the clinician is knowledgeable about the standards of care and is fully competent to apply those standards when caring for patients.[29]

Negligence is the failure to act in the required manner, causing harm to an individual. *Malpractice* is an unintentional act performed by a professional acting in a professional capacity that causes harm to an individual. Under the rule *respondeat superior* "let the master answer," an employer is held liable for acts of malpractice committed by an employee while performing duties for which she or he was hired.

For an action to fit the *legal definition of malpractice*, the following four elements must be met:

- *Duty:* The patient is owed a specific duty or standard of care.
- *Breach of duty:* There was a failure to meet the required standard of care.
- *Proximate cause:* A direct causal relationship exists between the breach of duty and the harm or injury to the patient.

- *Harm or injury:* Actual harm or injury occurred to the woman, fetus, or neonate as a result of the breach of duty.

Notification and Clinical Review

When there is error, injury, or other adverse outcome, there should be written and well-understood procedures to guide staff. Notification of supervisory or management-level individuals should be timely, according to organizational policy. Appropriate quality assurance memos or incident reports should be completed for performance improvement purposes. The medical record should contain documentation of the facts surrounding the event and should be free from editorial commentary and potentially damaging, biased, or blaming comments.

When an adverse outcome occurs, the entire perinatal unit is usually aware of the event. There is great interest in finding out what happened, and the staff sincerely wants to support the team members involved by reviewing the event in detail. However, chart review and questions in the absence of a "need to know" basis must be avoided. Any discussions occurring outside an official quality improvement or risk management forum will be discoverable in the event of litigation and can be required to be repeated under oath. Perinatal care providers should be knowledgeable about the appropriate time and place to discuss events, and they should be compliant with the Health Insurance Portability and Accountability Act regulations regarding protected patient information.

A critical incident debriefing by a skilled resource, such as an employee assistance program, a trained hospital-based team, a social worker, or a chaplain, provides an opportunity for staff to process feelings and concerns related to adverse outcomes and patient injuries in an environment free from discovery and blame. The critical incident debriefing is most effective when conducted as soon as possible after the occurrence of the event.

In the event of litigation, a plaintiff's attorney may attempt to make direct contact with nurses involved in the care of the allegedly injured patient. Hospital or unit orientation should include information about the correct response to such a request (refusal to discuss) and the requirement that the hospital's risk management department be notified and involved before any discussion with a plaintiff's attorney occurs (Box 10-4).

Reporting of Sentinel Events

Adverse events that meet the definition of a sentinel event (i.e., an unexpected occurrence involving death or serious physical or

---

BOX 10-4   Most Common Allegations of Obstetric Malpractice Claims

1. Failure to recognize or respond to changing fetal status
2. Failure to do a timely delivery
3. Failure to conduct proper resuscitation
4. Negligently causing vacuum or forceps injuries
5. Failure to prevent and manage shoulder dystocia
6. Improper use of oxytocin

Note: Absent or persistently minimal variability with recurrent late or variable decelerations or with bradycardia are associated with an increased risk of fetal metabolic acidemia.

psychologic injury, or the risk thereof) must be reported according to The Joint Commission and state department of health standards. A sentinel event signals the need for immediate investigation and response. The Joint Commission specifically lists "any intrapartum maternal death and any perinatal death unrelated to a congenital condition in an infant with birthweight >2500 grams" as voluntarily reportable events.[20] Following the report of a sentinel event, the organization must conduct a root-cause analysis and report the findings of that process to The Joint Commission. The root-cause analysis identifies causal factors for the sentinel event and improvements in processes or systems that would decrease the likelihood of such events in the future. Root-cause analysis follows an event and focuses primarily on systems and processes, not individual performance.

Failure Mode, Effect, and Criticality Analysis

In June 2001, The Joint Commission began requiring accredited hospitals to complete at least one yearly failure mode, effect, and criticality analysis (FMECA). An FMECA differs from a root-cause analysis in being a proactive, systematic examination of a process, such as fetal monitoring during labor, to identify ways in which failure *could* occur during the process. The assumption of the FMECA is that no matter how knowledgeable or careful people are, errors will occur and may even be *likely* to occur. Proactive identification of potential errors (failure modes) enables the organization to make changes in a process to prevent error and injury from occurring.[20]

DOCUMENTATION

Medico-legal risk management at its core involves communication, both written and verbal. The medical record and the terms utilized therein will be what attorneys, claim representatives, and reviewing expert physicians pre-judge. Furthermore, the accuracy of terms and the consistency of terminology among providers will weigh in judging not only the competency but also the credibility of providers.

To reduce risk, appropriate documentation must be kept, including the frequency of, content reviewed, and nomenclature utilized for fetal heart rate evaluation. Providers must know, understand, and utilize institutional policies, guidelines, and resources in the delivery of appropriate care and documentation. These documents will form either the shield of the provider's defense or the sword for the plaintiff.

Documentation in the patient's record is used to describe care and interventions provided in a sequential manner. This information may be stored or archived on an optical disk or other device (Figure 10-4). In some states, it is lawful to discard the paper strip once it is confirmed that all monitoring data are captured in the

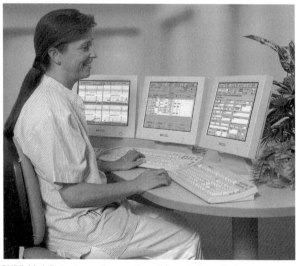

FIGURE 10-4 Data storage is an option with central monitoring systems. Information is stored on an optical disk and can be easily retrieved and printed in its original quality. A security system prevents the editing or addition of information to the stored data. (Courtesy Philips Medical Systems, Böblingen, Germany.)

electronic system. Increasing evidence indicates that documentation should be done only once, on the paper labor flow sheet or in the electronic record, to avoid duplication.[24] *Duplicative charting presents a significant risk of inconsistencies* that can be questioned or challenged by plaintiff attorneys in the event of future litigation. Furthermore, duplicative documentation in the medical record and on the fetal monitor strip is unnecessarily labor intensive for nurses who are frequently fully occupied in care of the woman and fetus.

To fully understand documentation issues in electronic fetal monitoring, the clinician must understand the difference between *assessment, communication*, and *documentation* (Figure 10-5). These are three distinct components of patient care, yet many nursing protocols fail to recognize the difference among these components, resulting in difficulty in compliance with documentation policies and excessive amounts of nursing time spent "nursing the chart" rather than providing patient care. A brief review is warranted here.

Components of Care: Assessment, Communication, Documentation

Assessment, the evaluation of patient status, is constant, ongoing, and very detailed. Clinicians notice many things about patients, not all of which are sufficiently clinically relevant to warrant communication or

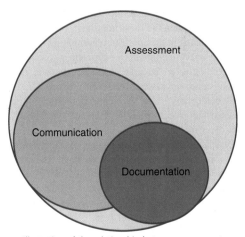

FIGURE 10-5 Illustration of the relationship between assessment, communication, and documentation in daily clinical practice. (Courtesy Lisa A. Miller, CNM, JD.)

documentation. Indeed, much of what a nurse assesses and many activities a nurse performs are never communicated to other providers nor do they appear in the medical record. Examples include the act of introducing oneself to the patient and family, changing a soiled gown or sheet, or simply offering support or encouragement to the patient and her family. *Thus the oft-quoted adage "if it wasn't charted, it wasn't done" has never been and will never be true.* Yet many clinicians readily agree with this statement when being deposed in relation to a malpractice suit. The reality is, there is absolutely no rationale, and it would not be physically possible, to either communicate or document all the assessments and activities of any clinician, whether nurse, midwife, or physician. Assessment is simply too broad a category.

Communication is slightly less broad but still encompasses more than any clinician can, or needs, to document. Much communication in labor and delivery is routine, consisting of sharing information or giving instructions to patients and family members. It may include notification of the charge nurse or team leader regarding status changes or patient updates, not all of which needs to be placed in the medical record. Notification of the midwife or physician regarding labor progress and fetal status may be quite detailed, but could be documented simply as "Provider updated as to patient status." There is no requirement, and it would not be effective use of a clinician's time, to document verbatim each and every conversation that occurs over the course of labor and birth.

Documentation, therefore, is the least broad of the three categories, and yet it is often the most important in relation to litigation. Evidence is presented in the courtroom in the form of exhibits or testimony. The primary exhibit in a malpractice case is the medical record. Accordingly, an accurate contemporaneous record is the foundation of either the plaintiff or defense case.

The best evidentiary friend of a plaintiff attorney is either inaccurate or inconsistent documentation of the care provided. Inaccurate documentation can stem from a competency issue, for example, where a fetal heart rate tracing is not appropriately interpreted, or from inaccurate nomenclature, such as what is present on the tracing. In either situation, the health care provider is left with a narrative note or deposition testimony which is inconsistent with the objective evidence on the tracing. Inconsistencies within a courtroom do not favor the inconsistent party.

Conflicting or contradictory documentation and use of nomenclature create difficulties for clinicians in both the screening and testimonial phases of malpractice litigation. When a file is being *initially* reviewed by plaintiff's counsel to determine whether or not medical malpractice may have occurred, the medical record is the only documentation available. The narrative note supplied will be read against subsequent health care providers' notes and a fetal heart rate tracing. Accurate recognition and description of fetal heart rate assessments in the patient's chart demonstrate attentive and competent care. Inaccurate or incorrect terminology in a medical record when read and compared with the objective fetal heart tracing increases the likelihood of litigation.

Compounding the matter further, *inconsistent and inaccurate nomenclature* also create difficult obstacles *later*, during the testimonial phase of litigation. When a witness uses modified or nonstandardized nomenclature, other health care providers and expert witnesses will not understand the full extent of what is meant. This creates unclear communication which can result in medical errors or the appearance of errors within a medical record. This problem is exemplified by the following deposition excerpt.

Deposition Excerpt # 1

A physician (MD) was questioned in deposition by the plaintiff's attorney (PA) regarding a nursing narrative note.

PA: Dr. Doe, do you expect an intrapartum nurse to relay to you if there is any late component to a deceleration?

MD: Any late decelerations should be relayed to me, particularly if there is more than one.

PA: By late deceleration do you mean if any portion of the deceleration is thought to be late?

MD: I do not understand what that means. However, if a nurse sees something late, I want to know about it immediately, especially if it recurs.

The narrative notes within the case included the nurse documenting variable decelerations with "late components." Utilizing the terminology "late components" created a scenario where the significance is undefined and suggests a call should have been made. Further testimony demonstrated that no information regarding this deceleration was relayed. The nurse testified as follows:

PA: Did you relay to Dr. Doe this deceleration had late components?

RN: No.

PA: Why not?

RN: Because I felt it was a variable deceleration with late components and was not nonreassuring.

PA: So you felt it was a variable and not a late?

RN: Yes.

PA: So when you chart the word *late*, you want the jury to
believe it doesn't mean late?

RN: I guess.

The inappropriate utilization of nomenclature has created a scenario
where the physician has inadvertently criticized the nurse. Furthermore, the nurse must separate herself from her own charting of the
word *late*. This makes the ability to defend the case more difficult.
With appropriate utilization of nomenclature, the nurse would have
simply charted this was a variable deceleration, which she did not
feel was recurrent, and it did not warrant immediate notification of
the physician given the clinical context.

The utilization of standardized nomenclature not only supports
the defense of a medical malpractice action, it more importantly
allows the physician and nurse to communicate clearly and make
certain they are accurately discussing the findings and placing the
same significance on each term.

Documentation Issues Specific to Electronic Fetal Monitoring

The National Institute of Child Health and Human Development
(NICHD) in 1997 published nomenclature which standardized the
language utilized in the interpretation of fetal heart tracings.[38]
Between 2005 and 2006 all professional organizations in the U.S.
adopted the NICHD terminology.[2,3,6] Unfortunately, despite the
attempts at standardization of nomenclature, many health care providers have been slow to adapt. This creates the risk of inaccurate communication between health care providers who misuse terms, and it
creates the potential for a medical record replete with inconsistencies.

There are several documentation issues that relate specifically to
electronic fetal monitoring. These include what should be included
in electronic fetal monitoring documentation, definition and use of
summary terms, further quantification of decelerations, and frequency of documentation versus frequency of assessment.

Each institution must address these issues and provide guidance
for staff members. There are few absolutes for any of these issues
and institutional approaches will naturally vary, but some general
principles will provide a starting point for team discussion.

Components of Electronic Fetal Monitoring Evaluation

The NICHD panel identified five components to be included in evaluation of the fetal heart rate tracing[38]:

- Baseline rate
- Baseline variability
- Presence of accelerations
- Periodic or episodic decelerations
- Changes or trends over time

These five components form the basis of electronic fetal monitoring management and should be included in documentation related to the fetal heart rate tracing. If using a graphic flowsheet, the fifth component (changes or trends over time) is apparent by simple review of the flowsheet. However, when clinicians use narrative charting, as is the case for most doctors and midwives, changes or trends over time may need to be specifically identified. In addition to the five fetal heart rate components, *documentation should include uterine activity and mode of assessment* (external or internal).

Use of Summary Terms *Reassuring* and *Nonreassuring*

One of the greatest problem areas in both documentation and deposition testimony is the use of summary terms, such as *reassuring* and *nonreassuring,* in relation to electronic fetal monitoring. Poorly defined in the literature, these terms continued to be used by many clinicians in both communication and documentation. Lack of specific or standardized definitions for their use leads to confusion and has potential for miscommunication. The following deposition excerpt illustrates the predicament.

Deposition Excerpt # 2

In a case where the plaintiff allegations included failure to perform a cesarean section for fetal distress, a physician (MD) was questioned in deposition by the plaintiff's attorney (PA) regarding definition of the term *nonreassuring*.

PA: Dr. Casey, what does a nonreassuring FHR tracing mean to you?

MD: It means I need to deliver the baby. It means the fetus cannot tolerate labor.

PA: And in this case was the tracing ever nonreassuring?

MD: Absolutely not. There were some decelerations but it never rose to the level of nonreassuring.

Unbeknownst to the physician, the nursing flowsheet had boxes for the nurse to check as to whether the fetal heart rate tracing was "reassuring" or "nonreassuring." Hospital protocol dictated the nurse must choose one of the terms; there was no third category or option for tracings that were "in between." The nurse testified as follows:

PA: Do you agree that part of what you do as a labor and delivery nurse is to identify a fetus at risk for asphyxia based on the fetal monitor tracing?

RN: I look at tracings and see whether they're reassuring or nonreassuring.

PA: And what is your definition for *reassuring* as it relates to a FHR tracing?

RN: A tracing that has two accelerations in 20 minutes.

PA: Is that in a laboring patient?

RN: Labor or no labor, that is what we expect.

PA: Do you still use the term *fetal distress*?

RN: No, that was years ago.

PA: Well, what does the term *fetal distress* mean to you?

RN: Well, it's like a nonreassuring heart rate. Something that was showing me the baby was not ... it would be a tracing that would not be reassuring me the baby was healthy. It could be variable or late decelerations, or a bradycardia.

PA: So today the word you would use instead of the term *fetal distress* is the word *nonreassuring*?

RN: Correct.

PA: And would you agree that if there were fetal distress the doctor should be notified?

RN: Yes, if it were a nonreassuring tracing; we don't use fetal distress.

Later in the deposition ...

PA: And just counting the boxes up on the flowsheet, Nurse Ames, how many times did you check the "nonreassuring" box under the FHR assessment in the 2 hours prior to delivery?

RN: I count six times.

PA: Did you notify the doctor about the nonreassuring tracing? [referring to the first incidence of the RN checking the "nonreassuring" box on the flowsheet]

RN: No.

PA: Why not?

RN: I didn't think it was that nonreassuring.

The physician and nurse had different ideas regarding the use of the terms *reassuring* and *nonreassuring*, making it appear that one of them was incorrect or missed something. The nursing flowsheet that forced the registered nurse to choose one of the two terms without providing clear definitions for either of the terms created both a communication problem and a perfect opportunity for the plaintiff's attorney to take advantage of what could appear to a jury to be significant differences in the nurse's and the physician's testimonies.

The use of poorly defined summary terms can lead to miscommunication and confusion at a minimum and may lead to medical-legal difficulties should clinicians find themselves involved in litigation. The easiest solution is simply to avoid the use of summary terms such as *reassuring* and *nonreassuring* and instead simply communicate using the five components of the fetal heart rate tracing: baseline rate, baseline variability, presence of accelerations, periodic or episodic decelerations, and changes or trends over time.[38] For institutions that decide to continue with the use of summary terms, standardized definitions should be collaboratively agreed upon and all clinicians should understand and be able to articulate those definitions. To that end, there are resources for coming to consensus regarding summary terms (Box 10-5).

The NICHD panel[38] did find agreement related to the summary term *normal*, which included a normal fetal heart rate baseline, moderate variability, presence of accelerations, and absence of decelerations. This definition could also be used for *reassuring*. At the other end of the continuum, the panel[38] and other experts[13] have noted that absent or persistently minimal variability, with recurrent late or variable decelerations or with bradycardia, have strong correlation with significant fetal acidemia. These patterns dictate preparation for delivery and may be appropriate to define *nonreassuring*. The conundrum arises with summary terms in clinical practice, when fetal heart rate patterns fall between the two ends of the spectrum. Fox and colleagues[13] described use of the term *variant* to apply to fetal heart rate

---

BOX 10-5   Use of Summary Terms – *Reassuring* and *Nonreassuring* Fetal Heart Rate and Preferred Documentation

Reassuring[38]
   Normal baseline rate
   Moderate variability
   Presence of accelerations
   Absence of decelerations
Nonreassuring[13,38]
   Absent or persistently minimal variability with recurrent late or variable decelerations or with bradycardia are associated with an increased risk of fetal metabolic acidemia.
Preferred Documentation, Based on Five Components of the FHR Tracing
   1. Baseline rate
   2. Baseline variability
   3. Presence of accelerations
   4. Periodic or episodic decelerations
   5. Changes or trends over time

patterns with moderate variability and tachycardia, bradycardia, or recurrent decelerations to differentiate them from both the NICHD's *normal* and the patterns associated with fetal acidemia. Unfortunately, the term *variant* as defined by Fox and colleagues does not account for a variety of patterns that do not meet any of the aforementioned categories, such as minimal variability that is not persistent or marked variability with tachycardia. Perhaps the term *variant* could be expanded, or an alternate term, such as *intermediate* could be used to incorporate all fetal heart rate tracings that fall on the continuum somewhere between normal/reassuring and the nonreassuring/indicative of fetal acidemia. As this discussion makes clear, institutions and clinicians need to exercise caution with regard to use of summary terms and may be smart in simply avoiding their use altogether.

Quantification of Decelerations

It should be noted that while the NICHD panel[38] discussed the option of further quantifying decelerations by duration (onset to offset) and depth of nadir, this was not a mandate. Given that early decelerations are not associated with hypoxemia, further quantification of early decelerations does not seem clinically indicated or logical. Late decelerations reflect transient hypoxemia and warrant a clinical response regardless of depth, making further quantification moot. However, management of variable and prolonged decelerations may differ based on duration and depth of nadir, making it reasonable to further quantify these decelerations at least in communication with the team members, especially if the recipient of the communication does not have visual access to the fetal heart rate tracing. Communication is distinct from documentation and is often more detailed than what is documented in the medical record, as discussed above. Institutions will need to decide whether further quantification of decelerations is warranted in documentation practices, and if so, whether it is necessary for all deceleration types.

Frequency of Electronic Fetal Monitoring Assessment Versus Frequency of Electronic Fetal Monitoring Documentation

As discussed earlier in this chapter, assessment encompasses a clinical spectrum that is much larger than just documentation. Frequency of fetal heart rate tracing assessment may vary both by stage of labor as well as clinical context (antepartum vs. intrapartum, risk factors, previous fetal heart rate tracing, interventions). When utilizing electronic fetal monitoring, a continuous permanent record is created and is often archived electronically in addition to (or as an alternative to) an actual paper strip. Institutional protocols should be in place to delineate both the frequency of assessment of fetal heart rate tracings as well as the frequency of documentation regarding fetal heart rate findings. It is reasonable that fetal heart rate assessments may be more frequent than fetal heart rate documentation, in keeping with the reality of clinical practice. While a detailed discussion of perinatal documentation policies is beyond the scope of this book, all documentation policies related to electronic fetal monitoring should address the following:

- Recognition of the difference between assessment, communication, and documentation
- The five components of FHR evaluation (baseline rate, baseline variability, presence of accelerations, periodic/episodic decelerations, changes/trends over time)
- Evaluation of uterine contractions (UC), including frequency, duration, and strength
- Frequency of FHR and UC evaluation/assessment
- Minimum frequency of documentation of FHR and UC findings
- Definitions of any summary terms, if utilized

It is imperative that institutions create reasonable and rational policies regarding all three areas: assessment, communication, and documentation. While there is no one "right" way to accomplish this, the principles discussed above should serve as a starting point for clinicians, regardless of specialty. Documentation practices and policies will vary reasonably, based on type of system (computerized records vs. paper), style of charting (flowsheet vs. narrative), clinical context (labor evaluation vs. non-labor complaint), and numerous other factors. Addressing the key issues above will result in the development of sound, clinically realistic policies in regard to documentation.

Electronic Medical Records and Information Systems

Computerized perinatal information systems are becoming more and more common as health care institutions strive to improve information flow and documentation practices. The options range from simple archiving of fetal heart rate tracings to completely integrated systems linking prenatal outpatient care to inpatient intrapartum and neonatal recordkeeping. Many systems offer remote viewing via computer intranet access, with at least one system offering data access, including real-time fetal heart rate tracing review, via mobile phone. Another system utilizes several onscreen tools that provide graphic overlays to help clinicians correctly apply the NICHD definitions and reach consensus regarding fetal heart rate tracing components (Figure 10-6). As compared to traditional paper records, *computerized systems offer several benefits,*[32,56] including the following:

- Single data entry for use on multiple forms/records
- Forced functions that promote user compliance with standardized terms and/or evaluations
- Ability to view information in several formats, such as timeline and graphic
- Automatic creation of notes and minimization of narrative/typing using preset scripts and drop-down menus
- Improved readability of records (avoidance of illegibility)
- Bedside access to protocols, policies, calculators, and other tools to improve or facilitate patient care
- Access to multiple patient screens or multiple FHR tracings at a single computer display
- Facilitated data management and retrieval for reporting, statistics, and quality assurance activities

While the popularity and acceptance of computerized perinatal information systems continues to grow, it is essential that institutions recognize the importance of appropriate training and an organized transition plan when moving from paper charting to electronic medical records. Setting a "go-live" date and providing adequate time for clinicians to become proficient with the system before that date are keys to a smooth transition. *Having clinicians "double-chart" over a transition period is a poor strategy,*[24] replete with error potential and frustration for clinicians who are already burdened with documentation and administrative duties in addition to patient care.

Finally, it is important to note that computerized medical record systems vary with regard to transparency regarding documentation timing. Most systems provide the option to have medical record printouts that include keystroke data (i.e., the time the note was actually typed or entered) adjacent to the timing of the note. This information is sometimes referred to as the history or audit trail. When this information is included in the medical record printouts, the medical record is considered to be "transparent," meaning that a reviewer is able to clearly see the actual time the notation was entered. Problems can arise when the medical record printout does not include this information and clinicians have entered data that would normally be considered a late entry but do not identify it as

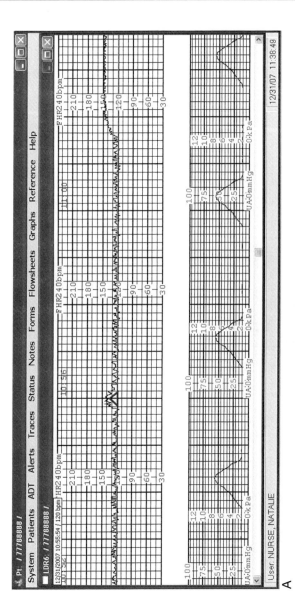

FIGURE 10-6 "E-tools" allow clinicians to confirm FHR findings based upon the NICHD terminology by overlaying them directly on the FHR tracing display on the computer. Pictured above is the Accel tool (**A**).

Continued

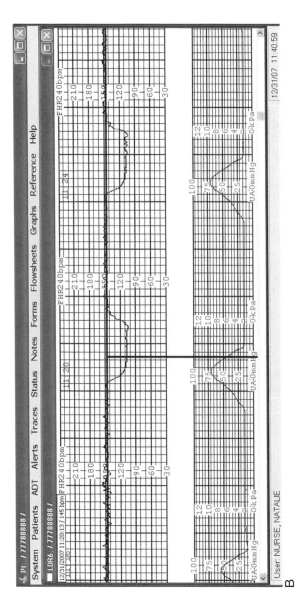

FIGURE 10-6 cont'd (B), The Decel tool allows users to measure the deceleration's onset to nadir and determine if it is abrupt (<30 sec) or gradual (≥30 sec). Other tools include tools for baseline rate and baseline variability. (Courtesy Clinical Computer Systems, Elgin, IL.)

such. If the computer printout of the medical record gives the appearance of contemporaneous charting, but the audit trail or history reveals the actual time of the entry was hours or days after the notation time, it could be construed as a clinician's attempt to "buff" the chart. This can result in allegations of spoliation in medical malpractice cases. *Spoliation* refers to the withholding or hiding of evidence in legal proceedings and could include additions to the medical record with the purpose of falsification to avoid liability. These allegations can be devastating to the defense of a medical malpractice suit. They are easily avoided by providing medical records that are transparent as to data entry and by setting reasonable standards for late entries and addendums to medical records.

Record Storage and Retrieval

The fetal monitor tracing is a part of the patient's medical record; therefore, storage, security, and record retrieval are the responsibility of the hospital's medical records department. If the paper strip is archived, each segment of the strip must be clearly identified per unit policy. The strips should be numbered sequentially and securely banded together for archiving. Confidentiality of the fetal monitor tracings must be maintained by storing them in a secure place until the woman's entire medical record is sent to the medical records department. A process must be in place to request and reliably retrieve all fetal monitoring tracings, whether on paper, microfilm, or electronic archival. In the event of litigation, any missing monitoring information makes a case difficult (if not impossible) to defend despite excellent care and complete compliance with established standards.

SUMMARY

Risk management in perinatal care involves intentional action and process to avoid errors and to prevent injury or harm to mother and fetus. A primary tenet of risk reduction is the adoption of a patient safety approach to risk reduction, where system analysis of risk and error has replaced blame and focus on individual behavior/error. There are specific perinatal risk reduction strategies related to use of electronic fetal monitoring. An environment rich in competent care providers who practice as a team, use the same terminology, avoid variances in practice, and have systems in place for timely clinical intervention supports the likelihood of that organization being one of high reliability. Operating within a safety framework that includes ongoing clinical comprehension, communication, and collaboration improves patient care and reduces opportunity for error.

In formulating strategies and creating guidelines for patient care and documentation, clinicians and health systems must acknowledge and understand the difference between assessment, communication, and documentation. All of these areas have potential for error, but an approach that respects the realities of clinical practice and makes patient safety the top priority serves both patients and clinicians. Documentation issues specific to electronic fetal monitoring must be addressed, and any terminology utilized must be clearly defined, understood, and used consistently by all team members. Information technology and computerized perinatal information systems can assist clinicians in meeting this challenge.

Finally, clinicians have a duty to disclose unanticipated outcomes. Disclosure should be accomplished by trained individuals and should include a discussion of any errors in an honest and forthright manner. Through the combination of a core philosophy of patient safety, collaborative care and teamwork, and direct and open disclosure practices, patients and families can be assured that health care systems are working successfully towards improved outcomes. And nurses, midwives, and doctors can effectively abide by the ancient wisdom of *primum non nocere,* "first do no harm."

References

1. American Academy of Pediatrics, American College of Obstetricians and Gynecologists: *Guidelines for perinatal care,* ed 6, Washington, DC, 2007, AAP, ACOG.

2. American College of Nurse-Midwives: *Standard nomenclature for electronic fetal monitoring, Position Statement 2006,* Silver Spring, MD, 2006, ACNM.

3. American College of Obstetricians and Gynecologists: Intrapartum fetal heart rate monitoring, ACOG *Practice Bulletin* no.70, *Obstet Gynecol* 106(6):1453-1461, 2005.

4. American College of Obstetricians and Gynecologists: Inappropriate use of the terms fetal distress and birth asphyxia, *Committee Opinion* no. 197, Washington, DC, 1998, ACOG.

5. American College of Obstetricians and Gynecologists: Disclosure and discussion of adverse events, *Committee Opinion* no. 380, Washington, DC, 2007, ACOG.

6. Association of Women's Health, Obstetric and Neonatal Nurses: *Changes to the FHMPP program.* Accessed August 22, 2005, from www.awhonn.org/awhonn/pg=873-2180-17530.

7. Association of Women's Health, Obstetric, and Neonatal Nurses: *Fetal heart monitoring: Principles and practices,* ed 3, Dubuque, IA, 2003, Kendall/Hunt.

8. Association of Women's Health, Obstetric and Neonatal Nurses: *Clinical competencies and education guide: Fetal surveillance in antepartum and intrapartum nursing practice*, ed 3, Washington, DC, 1998, AWHONN.

9. Becher J, Stenson B, Lyon A: Is intrapartum asphyxia preventable? *BJOG* 114(11):1442-1444, 2007.

10. Conway JB, Weingart SN: Organizational change in the face of highly public errors, I: the Dana-Farber Cancer Institute Experience, *AHRQ Perspectives on Safety* [serial online] May 2005. Accessed October 29, 2007, from www.webmm.ahrq.gov/perspective.aspx?perspectiveID=3.

11. Draycott T, Sibanda T, Owen L, Akande V, Winter C, Reading S, Whitelaw L: Does training in obstetric emergencies improve neonatal outcome? *BJOG* 113(2):177-182, 2006.

12. Forster AJ, O'Rourke K, Shojania KG, van Walraven C: Combining ratings from multiple physician reviewers helped to overcome the uncertainty associated with adverse event classification, *J Clin Epidemiol* 60(9): 892-901, 2007.

13. Fox M, Kilpatrick S, King, T, Parer J: Fetal heart rate monitoring interpretation and collaborative management, *J Midwifery Womens Health* 45(6): 498-507, 2000.

14. Gallagher T, Studdert D, Levinson W: Disclosing harmful medical errors to patients, *N Engl J Med* 356(26):2713-2719, 2007.

15. Gennaro S, Mayberry LJ, Kafulafula U: The evidence supporting nursing management of labor, *J Obstet Gynecol Neonatal Nurs* 36(6): 598-604, 2007.

16. Greenwald L, Mondor M: Malpractice and the perinatal nurse, *J Perinat Neonatal Nurs* 17(2):101-109, 2003.

17. Haig KM, Sutton S, Whittington J: SBAR: A shared mental model for improving communication between clinicians, *Jt Comm J Qual Patient Saf* 32(3):167-175, 2006.

18. Harris KT, Treanor CM, Salisbury ML: Improving patient safety with team coordination: challenges and strategies of implementation, *J Obstet Gynecol Neonatal Nurs* 35(4):557-566, 2006.

19. Institute of Medicine: *To err is human: Building a safer health system*, Washington, DC, 2000, National Academy Press.

20. Joint Commission on Accreditation of Healthcare Organizations: *Comprehensive manual for accreditation of hospitals*, Oak Brook, IL, 2003, The Joint Commission.

21. Joint Commission on Accreditation of Healthcare Organizations (The Joint Commission): *Preventing infant death during delivery* (Sentinel Event Alert no. 30), Oak Brook, IL, 2003, The Joint Commission.

22. Jonsson M, Nordén SL, Hanson U: Analysis of malpractice claims with a focus on oxytocin use in labour, *Acta Obstetricia et Gynecologica Scandanavica* 86(3):315-319, 2007.

23. Katzenbach JR, Smith DK: *The wisdom of teams*, Boston, 1993, Harvard Business School Press.

24. Kelly CS: Perinatal computerized patient record and archiving systems: Pitfalls and enhancements for implementing a successful computerized medical record, *J Perinat Neonatal Nurs* 12(4):1-14, 1999.

25. Klein RL, Bigley JA, Roberts KH: Organization culture in high reliability organizations: An extension, *Human Relations* 48(1):1-23, 1995.

26. Knox G, Simpson K, Garite T: High Reliability Perinatal Units: An approach to the prevention of patient injury and medical malpractice claims, *J Health Risk Manag* 19(2):24-32, 1999.

27. Koniak-Griffin D: Strategies for reducing the risk of malpractice litigation in perinatal nursing, *J Obstet Gynecol Neonatal Nurs* 28(3):291-299, 1999.

28. Leonard M, Graham S, Bonacrum D: The human factor: The critical importance of effective teamwork and communication in providing safe care, *Qual Saf Health* 13(Suppl 1):i85-i90, 2004.

29. Mahlmeister L: Legal implications of fetal heart assessment, *J Obstet Gynecol Neonatal Nurs* 29(5):517-526, 2000.

30. Mahlmeister L: Professional accountability and legal liability for the team leader and charge nurse, *J Obstet Gynecol Neonatal Nurs* 28(3): 300-309, 1999.

31. Mazza F, Kitchens J, Kerr S, Markovich A, Best M, Sparkman LP: Eliminating birth trauma at Ascension Health, *Jt Comm J Qual Patient Saf* 33(1):15-24, 2007.

32. McCartney PR: Using technology to promote perinatal patient safety, *J Obstet Gynecol Neonatal Nurs* 35(3):424-431, 2006.

33. McFerran S, Nunes J, Pucci D, Zuniga A: Perinatal patient safety project: A multicenter approach to improve performance reliability at Kaiser Permanente, *J Perinat Neonatal Nurs* 19(1):37-45, 2005.

34. McRae M: Fetal surveillance and monitoring: Legal issues revisited, *J Obstet Gynecol Neonatal Nurs* 28(3):310-319, 1999.

35. Miller LA: Patient safety and teamwork in perinatal care, *J Perinat Neonatal Nurs* 19(1):46-51, 2005.

36. Miller LA: System errors in intrapartum electronic fetal monitoring: A case review, *J Midwifery Womens Health* 50(6):507-517, 2005.

37. Miller LA: Safety promotion and error reduction in perinatal care: Lessons from industry, *J Perinat Neonatal Nurs* 17(2):128-138, 2003.

38. National Institute of Child Health and Human Development (NICHD) Research Planning Workshop: Electronic fetal heart rate monitoring: Research guidelines for interpretation, *Am J Obstet Gynecol* 177(6): 1385-1390, 1997.

39. National Patient Safety Foundation: *Talking to patients about health care injury: Statement of principle*, Chicago, 2000, NPSF.

40. Park K: Human error. In Salvendy G, editor: *Handbook of human factors and ergonomics*, New York, 1997, Wiley.

41. Queenan JT: Professional liability: Storm warning, *Obstet Gyn* 98(2): 194-197, 2001.

42. Raines D: Making mistakes: Prevention is key to error-free health care, *AWHONN Lifelines* 4(1):35-39, 2000.

43. Reason JT: Understanding adverse events: The human factor. In Vincent C, editor: *Clinical risk management*, London, 2001, BMJ Books.

44. Reeves M: Building expertise: Making the case for fetal heart monitoring certification, *AWHONN Lifelines* 5(2):71-72, 2001.

45. Roberts KH: Managing hazardous organizations, *California Management Review* 32(Summer):101-113, 1990.

46. Roberts KH: Some characteristics of high reliability organizations, *Organization Science* 1(2):160-177, 1990.

47. Rommal C: Risk management issues in the perinatal setting, *J Perinat Neonatal Nurs* 10(3):1-31, 1996.

48. Simpson KR: Measuring perinatal patient safety: Review of current methods, *J Obstet Gynecol Neonatal Nurs* 35(3):432-442, 2006.

49. Simpson KR: Failure to rescue: Implications for evaluating quality of care during labor and birth, *J Perinat Neonat Nurs* 19(1):24-34, 2005.

50. Simpson KR, Knox GE: Adverse perinatal outcomes: Recognizing, understanding, and preventing common accidents, *AWHONN Lifelines* 7(3):224-235, 2003.

51. Simpson KR, Knox GE: Common areas of litigation related to care during labor and birth: Recommendations to promote patient safety and decrease risk exposure, *J Perinat Neonatal Nurs* 17(2):94-109, 2003.

52. Simpson KR, Knox GE: Perinatal teamwork, *AWHONN Lifelines* 5(5):56-59, 2001.

53. Simpson KR, Knox GE: Risk management and EFM: Decreasing risk of adverse outcomes and liability exposure, *J Perinat Neonatal Nurs* 14(3):40-52, 2000.

54. Sinclair BP: Nurses and malpractice, *AWHONN Lifelines* 4(5):7, 2000.

55. Singh H, Thomas EJ, Petersen LA, Studdert DM: Medical errors involving trainees: A study of closed malpractice claims from 5 insurers, *Arch Intern Med* 167(19):2030-2036, 2007.

56. Slagle T: Perinatal information systems for quality improvement: Visions for today, *Pediatrics* 103(1 Suppl E):266-277, 1999.

57. Sleutel M, Schultz S, Wyble K: Nurses' views of factors that help and hinder their intrapartum care, *J Obstet Gynecol Neonatal Nurs* 36(3):203-211, 2007.

58. Veltman L: Poor systems create liability for good providers. In Garza M, Piver JS: *Ob-Gyn Malpract Prevent* 10(7):49-56, 2003.

59. White AA, Pichert JW, Bledsoe SH, Irwin C, Entman SS: Cause and effect analysis of closed claims in obstetrics and gynecology, *Obstet Gynecol* 105(5 Pt 1):1031-1038, 2005.

60. Young P, Hamilton R, Hodgett S, Moss M, Rigby C, Jones P, Johanson R: Reducing risk by improving standards of intrapartum fetal care, *J R Soc Med* 94(5):226-231, 2001.

Amnioinfusion

Amnioinfusion is the administration of room temperature isotonic solution such as normal saline or Ringer's lactate via a double-lumen intrauterine pressure catheter (IUPC) by either a gravity flow or an infusion pump to restore amniotic fluid volume. The procedure is intended to relieve intermittent umbilical cord compression that results in variable fetal heart rate decelerations and transient fetal hypoxemia. This procedure has no known impact on late decelerations, and is no longer recommended for dilution of meconium.

An amnioinfusion generally begins by administering a bolus of fluid (250 to 500 ml) over 20 to 30 minutes. The maintenance dose is infused at a rate of 2 to 3 ml/min (maximum of 180 ml/hr), during which time it is imperative that the amount of fluid returning is approximated and documented to avoid overdistention of the uterus. Assessment of the output can be accomplished by weighing the absorbent pads underneath the woman (1 ml = 1 g) and counting the number of pads changed. Assessment of uterine resting tone is also an important aspect of surveillance during the procedure, and it should not exceed 40 mm Hg. It is unlikely that more than 1000 ml of fluid need be administered, and if variable decelerations persist even after this amount of fluid has been instilled into the uterus, other therapies should be used as treatment. Iatrogenic polyhydramnios may cause a placental abruption or pressure on the maternal diaphragm causing shortness of breath, tachycardia, and a change in maternal blood pressure. A rapid release or "gush" of fluid predisposes the woman to a prolapsed umbilical cord. The preterm fetus may benefit from a warmed solution, thus avoiding bradycardia. A blood warmer is the safest method for administering warmed fluid. *The fluid should not be heated in a microwave or blanket warmer.* Warmed fluid is also suggested if the rate of the amnioinfusion exceeds 15 ml/min.

There are a variety of ways to perform an amnioinfusion. It is important that the institution has a policy and procedure in place and that they are followed.

INDICATIONS FOR AMNIOINFUSION

1. Laboring preterm women with premature rupture of the membranes (prophylactic)
2. Variable decelerations uncorrectable with conventional interventions
3. Significant oligohydramnios (amniotic fluid index ≤ 5) at term when labor is being induced

EQUIPMENT AND SUPPLIES

- Normal saline or Ringer's lactate solution, 1000 ml at room temperature
- Intrauterine catheter equipment, preferably with a double lumen and amnioport (if using single-lumen water-filled IUPC, intravenous [IV] extension tubing with twin sites or arterial line [12 inches] and a three-way stopcock are needed)
- Volumetric infusion pump and tubing, or IV pole for gravity flow
- Blood warmer or blood/fluid warming set (optional)

PROCEDURE

Amnioinfusion should be initiated after insertion of the intrauterine catheter. Before the procedure, the intrauterine resting tone should be noted with the woman in the right and left lateral and supine positions for later comparison. Various procedures have been discussed in the literature, and each institution determines its own obstetric policies and procedures. A sample procedure follows:

1. Connect the 1000-ml bottle of amnioinfusion solution to the IV tubing.
2. Flush the tubing with the solution.
3. Connect the tubing to the woman's IUPC via the amnioport or double-lumen IUPC, or via a three-way stopcock, depending on the type of IUPC used.
4. Initiate the flow of amnioinfusion and instill the initial bolus, usually 250 to 500 ml over a 20- to 30-minute period (10 to 15 ml/min) using either an infusion pump or gravity flow. If gravity flow is used, the solution must be hung about 3 to 4 feet above the level of the tip of the IUPC. If fluid will not run by gravity, check the position/placement of the IUPC.

5. When variable decelerations resolve, continue the infusion at a slower rate, usually about 2 to 3 ml/min (120 to 180 ml/hr), as ordered by the care provider. If variable decelerations are not relieved after infusing 800 to 1000 ml of solution, discontinue the procedure and perform an alternative intervention.

6. Observe and evaluate for amount and character of vaginal drainage. Vaginal output is assessed and documented to demonstrate that the volume infused is also coming back out and not causing overdistension of the uterus. Be vigilant for sudden "gushes" of fluid and assess for cord prolapse.

NOTE: Intrauterine resting tone will appear higher than normal, from 25 to 40 mm Hg, because of resistance to outflow through the tiny holes in the tip of the catheter. The true resting tone can be checked by temporarily discontinuing the flow of infusion.

PATIENT CARE

Care of the woman undergoing amnioinfusion includes the following:

1. Stop the infusion periodically, approximately every 30 to 60 minutes, to note the baseline uterine pressure. If the resting tone of the uterus exceeds 40 mm Hg, discontinue the infusion and notify the physician.

2. Change the underpads frequently to ensure the woman's comfort.

3. Note the color and amount of fluid on the underpads. The underpads may be weighed. Amounts of fluid returned should be determined (1 ml = 1 g).

4. Monitor for signs and symptoms of infection.

5. Monitor for signs and symptoms of cardiac or respiratory compromise secondary to an overexpanded uterus (maternal shortness of breath, hypotension, or tachycardia).

6. Monitor fetal heart rate patterns on the electronic fetal monitoring strip.

Selected Pattern Interpretations at 1 cm/min Paper Speed

Cardiotocography (electronic fetal heart rate [FHR] monitoring) outside of North America is usually done at a paper speed of 1 cm/min, which is slower than the 3 cm/min paper speed used in North America. Note that the fetal heart rate range is from 50 to 210 beats per minute (bpm) and that each vertical line on the trace paper is 30 seconds of time (Figure B-1).

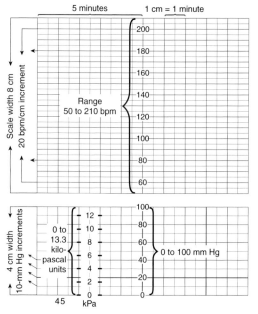

FIGURE B-1 Fetal monitor paper used in countries outside North America, with a paper speed of 1 cm/min.

REACTIVE FETAL HEART RATE ON ADMISSION

SIGNAL SOURCE	Spiral electrode and tocotransducer (1 cm/min)	
FHR	Baseline	120 to 130 bpm
	Variability	Moderate
	Periodic and episodic changes	Acceleration of FHR with uterine contractions and fetal movement
UTERINE ACTIVITY	Frequency	3½ to 4 minutes
	Duration	60 to 90 seconds

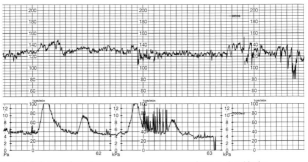

FIGURE B-2 1 cm/min (Courtesy Dr. Lennart Nordström, Stockholm, Sweden.)

REACTIVE NONSTRESS TEST

SIGNAL SOURCE	Ultrasound and tocotransducer (1 cm/min)	
FHR	Baseline	135 to 140 bpm
	Variability	Moderate
	Episodic changes	Accelerations of FHR

Baseline rate shows a quiet period without accelerations and baseline variability of 5 to 10 beats per minute followed by an active period indicated by fetal movement profile blocks. Note that there are more than two accelerations of more than 15 beats per minute lasting more than 15 seconds and an increase of variability.

Uterine Activity

Not in active labor

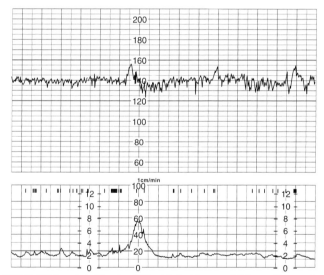

FIGURE B-3 1 cm/min (Courtesy Philips Medical Systems, Böblingen, Germany.)

NORMAL FETAL HEART RATE TRACING

SIGNAL SOURCE	Spiral electrode and IUPT* (1 cm/min)	
FHR	Baseline	132 bpm
	Variability	Moderate
	Episodic changes	Accelerations of FHR
UTERINE ACTIVITY	Frequency	2 to 3 minutes
	Duration	60 seconds
	Intensity	58 mm Hg
	Resting tone	15 mm Hg

*Intrauterine pressure transducer (same as IUPC).

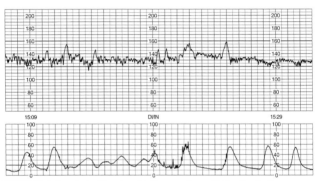

FIGURE B-4 1 cm/min (Courtesy Dr. Herman P. van Geijn, Amsterdam, The Netherlands.)

NORMAL TRACE OF FIRST STAGE OF LABOR

SIGNAL SOURCE	Ultrasound and tocotransducer (1 cm/min)	
FHR	Baseline	100 to 110 bpm
	Variability	Moderate
	Episodic changes	Acceleration of FHR with fetal movement
UTERINE ACTIVITY	Frequency	3 to 4 minutes
	Duration	60 seconds

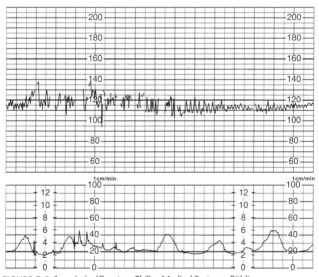

FIGURE B-5 1 cm/min (Courtesy Philips Medical Systems, Böblingen, Germany.)

UTERINE HYPERTONIA

SIGNAL SOURCE	Spiral electrode and IUPT (1 cm/min)	
FHR	Baseline	130 bpm
	Variability	Moderate
	Periodic changes	None
UTERINE ACTIVITY	Frequency	1 to 2 minutes
	Duration	60 seconds
	Intensity	50 to 60 mm Hg
	Resting tone	5 to 10 mm Hg

Note increase in resting tone with clustering of frequent uterine contractions.

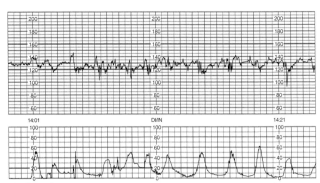

FIGURE B-6 1 cm/min (Courtesy Dr. Herman P. van Geijn, Amsterdam, The Netherlands.)

FLUCTUATING BASELINE/VARIABLE DECELERATIONS

SIGNAL SOURCE	Spiral electrode and tocotransducer (1 cm/min)	
FHR	Baseline	Fluctuating
	Variability	Moderate
	Episodic changes	Variable decelerations
UTERINE ACTIVITY	Frequency	2 to 3½ minutes
	Duration	60 to 90 seconds

This patient was a primigravida at 9 cm with a prolonged second stage. Fetal blood sampling revealed a pH of 7.25 and a lactate of 2.8 mmol/L (within normal limits).

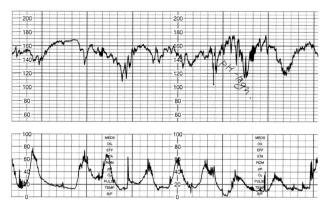

FIGURE B-7 1 cm/min (Courtesy Dr. Lennart Nordström, Stockholm, Sweden.)

SINUSOIDAL PATTERN

SIGNAL SOURCE	Ultrasound and tocotransducer (1 cm/min)	
FHR	Baseline	180 bpm— tachycardia
	Variability	Sinusoidal pattern
	Periodic/episodic	None
	Fetus had severe anemia.	
UTERINE ACTIVITY	Not in active labor; note the characteristic zigzag maternal respiratory movements on the uterine activity tracing.	

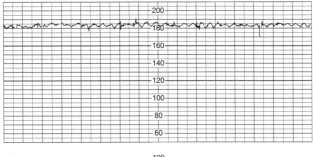

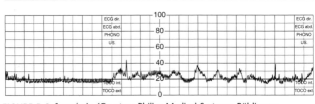

FIGURE B-8 1 cm/min (Courtesy Philips Medical Systems, Böblingen, Germany.)

TACHYCARDIA

SIGNAL SOURCE	Spiral electrode and IUPT (1 cm/min)	
FHR	Baseline	165 bpm
	Variability	Moderate
	Episodic changes	Accelerations and mild variable decelerations
UTERINE ACTIVITY	Frequency	1½ to 2 minutes
	Duration	60 seconds
	Intensity	Unable to determine exactly; approximately 40 to 50 mm Hg
	Resting tone	Unable to determine exactly; approximately 5 to 10 mm Hg

It does not appear that the UA was zeroed before use.

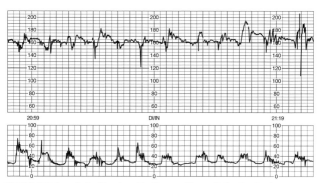

FIGURE B-9 1 cm/min (Courtesy Dr. Herman P. van Geijn, Amsterdam, The Netherlands.)

EARLY DECELERATIONS

SIGNAL SOURCE	Spiral electrode and tocotransducer (1 cm/min)	
FHR	Baseline	120 bpm
	Variability	Moderate
	Periodic changes	Early decelerations
UTERINE ACTIVITY	Frequency	4 to 5 minutes
	Duration	90 seconds

Note the mirror image of the early decelerations with the uterine contractions.

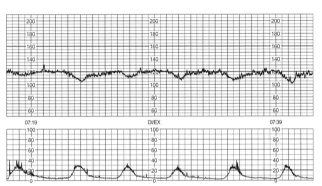

FIGURE B-10 1 cm/min (Courtesy Dr. Herman P. van Geijn, Amsterdam, The Netherlands.)

LATE DECELERATIONS

SIGNAL SOURCE	Spiral electrode and IUPT (1 cm/min)	
FHR	Baseline	165 bpm
	Variability	Moderate
	Periodic	Repetitive late
	changes	decelerations

Note that the nadir of the deceleration follows the peak of the uterine contraction.

UTERINE ACTIVITY	Frequency	2 to 4 minutes
	Duration	45 to 60 seconds
	Intensity	70 mm Hg
	Resting tone	15 mm Hg

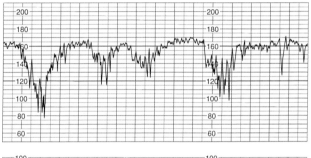

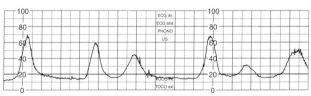

FIGURE B-11 1 cm/min (Courtesy Philips Medical Systems, Böblingen, Germany.)

MILD VARIABLE DECELERATIONS

SIGNAL SOURCE	Spiral electrode and IUPT (1 cm/min)	
FHR	Baseline	135 to 140 bpm
	Variability	Moderate
	Episodic	Mild variable
	changes	decelerations
UTERINE	Frequency	2 minutes
ACTIVITY	Duration	45 to 60 seconds
	Intensity	80 mm Hg
	Resting tone	5 to 10 mm Hg

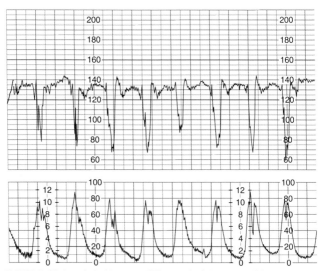

FIGURE B-12 1 cm/min (Courtesy Philips Medical Systems, Böblingen, Germany.)

VARIABLE DECELERATIONS

SIGNAL SOURCE	Spiral electrode and IUPT (1 cm/min)	
FHR	Baseline	140 to 150 bpm
	Variability	Moderate
	Episodic changes	Mild to moderate variable decelerations
UTERINE ACTIVITY	Frequency	2 to 3 minutes
	Duration	60 to 90 seconds
	Intensity	60 to 80 mm Hg
	Resting tone	15 to 20 mm Hg

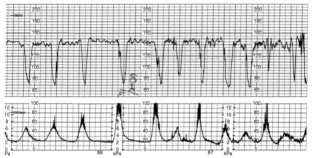

FIGURE B-13 1 cm/min (Courtesy Dr. Lennart Nordström, Stockholm, Sweden.)

VARIABLE DECELERATIONS

SIGNAL SOURCE	Spiral electrode and tocotransducer (1 cm/min)	
FHR	Baseline	140 to 150 bpm
	Variability	Moderate
	Episodic changes	Variable decelerations
UTERINE ACTIVITY	Frequency	2 to 3½ minutes
	Duration	60 to 90 seconds

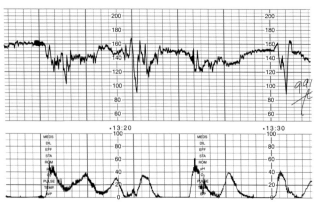

FIGURE B-14 1 cm/min (Courtesy Dr. Lennart Nordström, Stockholm, Sweden.)

MODERATE/SEVERE VARIABLE DECELERATIONS

SIGNAL SOURCE	Spiral electrode and tocotransducer (1 cm/min)	
FHR	Baseline	160 bpm (it was 140 bpm earlier in labor) progressing to unstable baseline FHR
	Variability	Moderate with episode of decreasing variability, slow return to baseline, and overshoot with some decelerations
	Episodic changes	Moderate to severe variable decelerations; note the shapes of the decelerations in the U, V, and W shapes characteristic of variable decelerations. Most of the decelerations last 60 seconds; the W-shaped decelerations, however, last appreciably longer.
UTERINE ACTIVITY	Frequency	2 to 4 minutes
	Duration	About 60 to 90 seconds

It is difficult to assess uterine activity in the first panel; this may be due to location of the tocotransducer and patient movement.

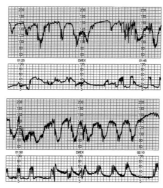

FIGURE B-15 1 cm/min (Courtesy Dr. Herman P. van Geijn, Amsterdam, The Netherlands.)

AMNIOINFUSION FOR VARIABLE DECELERATIONS

SIGNAL SOURCE	Spiral electrode and IUPT (1 cm/min)	
FHR	Baseline	Unstable initially, changing to 120 bpm after amnioinfusion
	Variability	Moderate to marked
	Episodic changes	Variable decelerations
		Note the progression to a severe variable deceleration that was immediately relieved by the amnioinfusion bolus of 500 ml of fluid.
UTERINE ACTIVITY	Frequency	2 to 3 minutes
	Duration	60 to 90 seconds
	Intensity	60 mm Hg
	Resting tone	20 mm Hg

It does not appear that the uterine activity baseline was zeroed before implementation of cardiotocography.

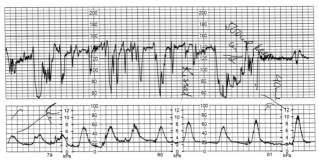

FIGURE B-16 1 cm/min (Courtesy Dr. Lennart Nordström, Stockholm, Sweden.)

PROLONGED DECELERATION SECONDARY TO UTERINE HYPERSTIMULATION

SIGNAL SOURCE	Spiral electrode and IUPT (1 cm/min)	
FHR	Baseline	140 bpm
	Variability	Moderate to marked
	Episodic changes	Prolonged deceleration
UTERINE ACTIVITY	Frequency	1½ to 2 minutes
	Duration	60 to 90 seconds
	Intensity	70 mm Hg
	Resting tone	20 mm Hg, increasing to 40 mm Hg before intervention

Oxytocin was discontinued immediately when hypertonus was observed but without effect on UA and fetal heart rate. A bolus of IV terbutaline (0.25 mg in 5 ml [indicated by the *arrow*]) relaxed the uterus within 2 minutes, and the fetal heart rate pattern returned to normal.

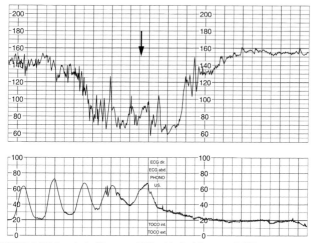

FIGURE B-17 1 cm/min (Courtesy Philips Medical Systems, Böblingen, Germany.)

GLOSSARY OF TERMS AND ABBREVIATIONS

abruptio placentae premature separation of the placenta before delivery of the fetus

acceleration transient increase in the fetal heart rate (FHR)

acidemia increased concentration of hydrogen ions in the blood

acidosis an increased concentration of hydrogen ions in tissue

AFI amniotic fluid index

amniocentesis procedure in which amniotic fluid is removed from the uterine cavity by insertion of a needle through the abdominal and uterine walls into the amniotic sac

amnioinfusion replacement of amniotic fluid with normal saline through an intrauterine pressure catheter

amnion inner of the two fetal membranes forming the sac that encloses the fetus within the uterus

amniotomy artificial rupture of the amniotic sac

anencephaly absence of the cerebrum, cerebellum, and flat bones of the skull

anoxia a total lack of oxygen in the tissue

Apgar score quantitative estimate of the condition of an infant at 1 and 5 minutes after birth, derived by assigning points to the quality of heart rate, respiratory effort, color, muscle tone, and response to stimulation; expressed as the sum of these points with the maximum score being 10

AROM artificial rupture of membranes

artifact irregularities on a fetal monitor tracing caused by electrical interference or poor reception of the FHR signal; may appear as scattered dots or lines

ASAP as soon as possible

AST acoustic stimulation test; same as vibroacoustic stimulation test, also known as fetal acoustic stimulation test, or FAST

AV atrioventricular

atelectasis collapse of the alveoli, or air sacs, of the lungs

augmentation correcting of ineffective uterine contractions (caused by dystocia) that occur after the start of spontaneous labor

baroreceptor a pressure receptor; a nerve ending located in the walls of the carotid sinus and the aortic arch that is sensitive to stretching induced by changes in blood pressure

base deficit a measure of the amount of base buffer reserves below normal levels; insufficient base buffer to buffer acids; expressed as a positive number (e.g., 12 mEq/L)

base excess a measure of the amount of base buffer reserves above normal levels; expressed as a negative number (e.g., -12 mEq/L); same as base deficit, but number is expressed as a negative number rather than as a positive number (i.e., base excess of -12 mEq/L is the same as base deficit of 12 mEq/L)

bilirubin pigment produced by the breakdown of hemoglobin in cell elements and in red blood cells

biparietal diameter distance from one parietal eminence to another; can be measured by ultrasound

BP blood pressure

bpm beats per minute

BPP biophysical profile

bradycardia baseline FHR below 110 bpm for 10 minutes

cardiotocography another term for electronic FHR monitoring

C/C/+1 used to indicate results of vaginal examination (e.g., cervix completely effaced/completely dilated/+1 station)

cephalopelvic disproportion (CPD) disparity between the size of the fetal head and the maternal pelvis, preventing vaginal delivery

cerebral palsy chronic static neuromuscular disability characterized by aberrant control of movement or posture

cervical ripening a complex process that culminates in the physical softening and distensibility of the cervix

chain of communication a reporting mechanism to resolve conflicts that threaten the quality or safety of patient care

chemoreceptor sensory end organ capable of reacting to a chemical stimulus

chorion outer of the two membranes forming the sac that encloses the fetus within the uterus

chromosome a dark-stained body within the cell nucleus that carries hereditary factors (genes); there are 46 chromosomes in each cell except in the mature ovum and sperm, where that number is halved

circumvallate placenta placenta in which an overgrowth of the decidua separates the placental margin from the chorionic plate, producing a thick, white ring around the circumference of the placenta and a reduction in distribution of fetal blood vessels to the placental periphery

CIS clinical information system; networked computer technologies that process patient information including data collection, alerting, documentation, analysis, storage, and retrieval

cm   centimeter

CMV   cytomegalovirus

CNS   central nervous system

coupling   two uterine contractions, one right after the other; the interval of time between the coupled contractions is less than the interval to the next uterine contraction or next set of coupled contractions

CP   cerebral palsy

CRP   C-reactive protein

CST   contraction stress test

CT   computed tomography

CTG   cardiotocography; another term for electronic FHR monitoring

CVS   chorionic villus sampling

deceleration   a decrease in the FHR; often occurs in response to a uterine contraction

DIL   cervical dilation

Doppler ultrasound   type of ultrasound that is reflected from moving interfaces, such as closure of fetal heart valves; Doppler ultrasound is used in electronic FHR monitors

DTR   deep tendon reflex

DW   dextrose in water

ECG   electrocardiogram

EDC   expected date of confinement

EFF   effacement of the cervix

effleurage   gentle stroking of the abdomen; used during labor in the Lamaze method of prepared childbirth

EFM   electronic fetal monitor(ing)

epidural   area situated on or over the dura mater; regional anesthetic is often injected into the peridural (epidural) space of the spinal cord

episodic changes   changes in the FHR that are not related to uterine contractions

extraovular   outside the amniotic fluid space (between the chorionic membrane and the endometrial lining)

FAST   fetal acoustic stimulation test

FBM   fetal breathing movements

FECG   fetal electrocardiogram

FGR   fetal growth restriction (replaces the term IUGR- intrauterine growth restriction)

FHR   fetal heart rate

FHT   fetal heart tones

FM   fetal movement

FMP   fetal movement profile

frequency (of contractions)   time from the onset of one uterine contraction to the onset of the next

FT   fetal tone

GBS   group B streptococcus

gestation   pregnancy; the period of intrauterine fetal development from conception to birth

gestational age   age of a conceptus computed from the first day of the last menstrual period to any point in time thereafter

HELLP syndrome   a disease characterized by hemolysis (H), elevated liver enzymes (EL), and low platelets (LP)

HR   heart rate

hydramnios   excessive volume of amniotic fluid, usually greater than 1.2 L; it is frequently seen in diabetic pregnancies and in fetuses with open neural tube defects (used interchangeably with polyhydramnios)

hydrocephaly   increased accumulation of cerebrospinal fluid within the ventricles of the brain; may result from congenital anomalies, infection, injury, or brain tumor; the head is usually large and globular with a disproportionately small face; the increased head diameter is possible in the fetus and infant because the sutures of the skull have not closed

hydrostatic pressure   pressure created in a fluid system

hyperthermia   hyperpyrexia; high fever

hypertonic   solution with a high osmotic pressure

hypertonus of the uterus   excessive muscular tonus or tension; abnormally high uterine resting tone

hypothermia   subnormal temperature of the body

hypotonic   solution with a low osmotic pressure

hypoxemia   decreased oxygen content in the blood

hypoxia   a decreased level of oxygen in tissue

hypoxic-ischemic encephalopathy   a subtype of neonatal encephalopathy for which the etiology is considered to be limitation of oxygen and blood flow near the time of birth

induction of labor   stimulation of uterine contractions before the spontaneous onset of labor for the purpose of accomplishing delivery

infant mortality   the number of deaths of infants under 1 year of age per 1000 live births in a given population per year

intervillous space   space between the myometrium and placental villi that is filled with maternal blood

intrapartum   occurring during labor or delivery

IUGR   intrauterine growth restriction (preferred term is now FGR-fetal growth restriction)

IUP   intrauterine pregnancy

IUPC   intrauterine pressure catheter

IUPT   intrauterine pressure transducer

IV   intravenous (parenteral fluids)

IVP   intravenous pyelogram

L   liter

laboring down   passive descent of the fetal head in the birth canal by uterine contractions (rather than active pushing) in the second stage of labor (after complete cervical dilation), until the woman experiences a strong urge to push; benefits include decreased use of instrumental delivery, decrease in duration of second stage of labor, decreased maternal fatigue, decreased incidence of second- and third-degree lacerations and episiotomies. Also known as "rest & descend," or "passive descent."

LATS   long-acting thyroid-stimulating hormone

LDR   labor/delivery/recovery room

L/S   lecithin-to-sphingomyelin ratio

macrosomia   large body size as seen in some postmature infants and in those born to diabetic mothers

MECG   maternal electrocardiogram

meconium   pasty greenish mass that collects in the fetal intestine, usually expelled during the first 3 to 4 days after birth; its presence in amniotic fluid may be of concern at the time of delivery should it be aspirated by the fetus; fetal naso-oropharynx is suctioned prior to delivery of the fetal body to avoid aspiration and resulting meconium aspiration syndrome

MHR   maternal heart rate

min   minutes

ml   milliliter

mm Hg   millimeters of mercury (unit of measure of pressure)

morbidity   the number of sick persons or cases of disease in relationship to a specific population

mortality   the death rate; the ratio of number of deaths to a given population

MRI   magnetic resonance imaging

MSpO$_2$ maternal oxygen saturation measured by pulse oximetry

mU   milliunits (used for oxytocin dosage, for example)

MVU   Montevideo unit

MW   molecular weight

nadir   the lowest point of a curve; the depth or trough of a FHR deceleration

NBP   maternal noninvasive blood pressure

neonatal encephalopathy   a clinically defined syndrome of disturbed neurologic function in the earliest days of life in the term infant, manifested by difficulty with initiating and maintaining respiration, depression of tone and reflexes, subnormal level of consciousness, and, often, seizures

NS   normal saline

NST   nonstress test

nuchal   neck (as in umbilical cord around the fetal neck)

OCT   oxytocin challenge test

OD   optical density

osmolality   quantity of a solute existing in solution as molecules or ions or both; the concentration of a solution

osmotic pressure   pressure developed when two solutions of the same solute at different concentrations are separated by a membrane permeable to the solvent only

P   pulse

p   statistical significance

peak   the highest point of a uterine contraction or FHR acceleration

periodic changes   changes in the FHR that are associated with uterine contractions, such as early and late decelerations

PG   phosphatidylglycerol

PI   phosphatidylinositol

placenta previa   placenta covering the internal cervical os

PMI   point of maximum intensity

PO   by mouth

polyhydramnios   *see* hydramnios (terms used interchangeably)

prn   as necessary

PROM   premature rupture of membranes

PTL   preterm labor

resting tone   intrauterine pressure between contractions (tonus)

R/O   rule out; consider as a possibility

ROM   rupture of membranes

SA   sinoatrial

sec   seconds

SGA   small for gestational age

SROM   spontaneous rupture of membranes

STA   station

supine hypotension syndrome   weight and pressure of uterus on the ascending vena cava when the patient is in a supine position decreases venous return, cardiac output, and blood pressure

surfactant   phospholipid that normally lines the alveolar sacs after 34 weeks of gestation. Its presence prevents collapse (atelectasis) of the alveoli by permitting a small amount of air to remain in the alveoli on exhalation. The L/S ratio is a measure of the presence of surfactant in amniotic fluid. Neonates born without surfactant develop respiratory distress syndrome (RDS).

tachycardia   baseline FHR above 160 bpm

tachysystole   excessive uterine contraction frequency; may occur with or without uterine stimulants

toco   tocotransducer or tocodynamometer, an external device used to record uterine activity

tocodynamometer   pressure-sensing instrument for measuring the duration and frequency of uterine contractions (used interchangeably with tocotransducer)

tocolytics   drugs used to inhibit uterine contractions and stop labor

tocotransducer   *see* tocodynamometer (terms used interchangeably)

tonus   intrauterine pressure between contractions (resting tone)

transducer   device that converts energy from one form to another; sound or pressure can be converted into an electrical impulse and vice versa

UA   uterine activity

UC   uterine contraction

ultrasound transducer   instrument that uses high-frequency sound (ultrasound) to detect moving interfaces, such as the closure of fetal heart valves, to monitor the FHR

US   ultrasound

variability   irregular fluctuations in the baseline FHR

VAS   vibroacoustic stimulation

VBAC   vaginal birth after cesarean

VDRL   Venereal Disease Research Laboratories

VE   vaginal examination

f indicates illustrations, b indicates boxes, and t indicates tables

Decelerations (*Continued*)
prolonged, 123–125
causes of, 124, 125
definition of, 97*b*, 123–124, 124*f*
fetal bradycardia and, 106
fetal oxygenation and, 124
interpretation of, 124–125
secondary to uterine
hyperstimulation,
interpretation of,
at 1cmm/min paper
speed, 265*f*, 265
qualification of, 236
variable, 121–123
amnioinfusion for, interpretation
of, at 1cm/min paper
speed, 264, 264*f*
atypical, 129–132
causes of, 121–123, 123
definition of, 97*b*, 121, 121*f*
fetal oxygenation and, 121–123
fluctuating, interpretation of,
at 1cm/min paper
speed, 255, 255*f*
interpretation of, 121–123
at 1cm/min paper speed, 261,
261*f*, 262, 262*f*
with late component, 130–131,
131*f*
mild, 131–132
interpretation of, at 1cm/min
paper speed, 260, 260*f*
moderate, 131–132
interpretation of, at 1cm/min
paper speed, 263, 263*f*
with overshoot, 129–130, 130*f*
severe, 131–132
interpretation of, at 1cm/min
paper speed, 263, 263*f*
shoulder in, 121–123, 127, 127*f*
"V-shaped,", 132, 133*f*
"W-shaped,", 132, 133*f*
DeLee-Hillis fetoscope, 28, 29*f*, 30
Delivery
"decision to" time, in managing
intrapartum fetal heart
rate, 144*t*, 149–151
rapid, clearing obstacles to, in
managing intrapartum fetal
heart rate, 144*t*, 148–149
vaginal, time until, 149

Diffusion
facilitated, in exchange between
maternal and fetal
blood, 17*t*
simple, in exchange between fetal
and maternal blood, 17*t*
Documentation, 227–241
of auscultated fetal heart rate, 33
as component of care, 229*f*, 230
conflicting or contradictory, 230
electronic fetal monitoring,
232–237
frequency of, versus frequency
of electronic fetal
monitoring assessment,
236–237
electronic medical records for,
237–241
Doppler ultrasound devices, 2
in fetal heart rate monitoring, 28
Doppler velocimetry, umbilical
artery, in antepartum
assessment, 203
Duty
breach of, as element of
malpractice, 225
as element of malpractice, 225
Dyskinetic cerebral palsy, hypoxic-
ischemic injury and, 25
Dysmaturity, in postterm
pregnancy, 172
Dystocia
cesarean deliveries due to, 85
risk of, decreasing, 85

E

Education, joint nurse/provider, in risk
reduction, 223
EFM. *See* Electronic fetal monitoring
(EFM).
Electrode, spiral, for fetal heart rate
monitoring, 35. *See also*
Spiral electrode, for fetal
heart rate monitoring.
Electronic fetal monitoring (EFM), 2
assessment of, frequency of, versus
frequency of electronic
fetal monitoring
documentation, 236–237